SORROW BUILT A BRIDGE
Friendship and AIDS

Daniel Berrigan, S.J.

WIPF & STOCK · Eugene, Oregon

Wipf and Stock Publishers
199 W 8th Ave, Suite 3
Eugene, OR 97401

Sorrow Built a Bridge
Friendship and AIDS
By Berrigan, Daniel
Copyright©1989 Catholic Worker Books
ISBN 13: 978-1-60608-469-4
Publication date 4/2/2009
Previously published by Fortkamp Publishing Company, 1989

To the Beloved Healers of the Supportive Care Program

Betsy
Graham
Cathy
Bill
Carole
Ed
Kathleen
Sr. Pat
Sr. Jorene
Jane
Paulette
Sr. Patrice
Cynthia
Sheryl
Patty

. . . .
If one suffers, all suffer
If one is honored, all rejoice

SERIES FOREWORD

Daniel Berrigan is one of the most influential American Catholics of the twentieth century. A Jesuit priest, poet, and peacemaker, he has inspired countless people of faith and conscience to pursue the gospel vision of a world without war or nuclear weapons. Born in 1921, he entered the Society of Jesus in 1939, was ordained in 1952, and in 1957 published his first book of poetry, *Time Without Number*, which won the prestigious Lamont Poetry Award.

Since then Daniel Berrigan, my friend and Jesuit brother, has published over fifty books, including the award-winning play, *The Trial of the Catonsville Nine* (1970); an autobiography, *To Dwell in Peace* (1987); and many journals, essays, poetry collections, and scripture commentaries. Dan maintained close friend friendships with Thomas Merton and Dorothy Day. He also co-founded the Catholic Peace Fellowship and Clergy and Laity Concerned about Vietnam. But because of his early peace work, church authorities banished him to Latin America in 1966 and 1967. In early 1968, he traveled to Hanoi with Howard Zinn to experience firsthand the horrors of U.S. war-making and to rescue three U.S. soldiers who had been captured.

On May 19, 1968, with his brother Philip and other friends, he burned military draft files using homemade napalm in Catonsville, Maryland—an action which galvanized millions against the Vietnam war. For this creative nonviolence, Dan was tried, convicted, and sentenced to years in prison. In April of 1970, however, he went underground, eluding the FBI, and continued to draw widespread attention to his antiwar message. He was finally arrested in August, and imprisoned in Danbury, Connecticut until February 1972.

He continued to write and speak against war and nuclear weapons throughout the 70s. On September 9, 1980, both he and Philip participated in the first Plowshares Action, a protest at the General Electric Plant at King of Prussia, Pennsylvania. He faced ten years in prison, but was eventually sentenced to time served.

Since the early 1970s, Dan has lived in New York City with his Jesuit community. He continues to give lectures, conduct retreats, publish books of poetry and scripture study—and get arrested for his protests against war, injustice, and nuclear weapons. He remains a clear voice of resistance to war, gospel nonviolence, and peace for humanity.

Throughout his faithful, peacemaking life, Daniel Berrigan has consistently said no to every war, injustice, and weapon of violence. And with every no he accepts the cost. And he does not give up. Nominated many times for the Nobel Peace Prize, Dan often finds himself with friends before some judge and sitting on ice in some dismal holding cell. Such is the mark of a prophet, the sign of an apostle of peace.

"We have assumed the name of peacemakers," Dan writes in *No Bars to Manhood*,

> but we have been, by and large, unwilling to pay any significant price. And because we want the peace with half a heart and half a life and will, the war, of course, continues, because the waging of war, by its nature, is total—but the waging of peace, by our own cowardice, is partial. There is no peace because there are no peacemakers. There are no makers of peace because the making of peace is at least as costly as the making of war, at least as exigent, at least as disruptive, at least as liable to bring disgrace and prison and death in its wake.

Foreword

"The only message I have to the world is: we are not allowed to kill innocent people," he told the court during his Plowshares Eight trial.

> We are not allowed to be complicit in murder. We are not allowed to be silent while preparations for mass murder proceed in our name, with our money, secretly. . . . It's terrible for me to live in a time where I have nothing to say to human beings except, 'Stop killing.' There are other beautiful things that I would love to be saying to people. There are other projects I could be very helpful at. And I can't do them. I cannot. Because everything is endangered. Everything is up for grabs. Ours is a kind of primitive situation, even though we would call ourselves sophisticated. Our plight is very primitive from a Christian point of view. We are back where we started. 'Thou shalt not kill'; we are not allowed to kill. Everything today comes down to that—everything.

I am very grateful to Wipf and Stock Publishers for republishing some of Dan's classic works in a series, books which influenced millions of people when they first appeared. I hope these books will be studied, passed around to friends and neighbors, and promoted far and wide. They still offer great hope, wisdom, and encouragement.

In the life and words of Daniel Berrigan we discover new faith in the God of peace and courage to pursue God's reign of peace. We see signs and guideposts for the path ahead, toward a new future of peace. And we find strength to take our own stand for justice and disarmament, to take another step forward on the road to peace and nonviolence. May these books inspire us to become, like Daniel Berrigan, peacemakers in a world of war.

—John Dear
Cerrillos, New Mexico
August 2007

SORROW BUILT A BRIDGE
Friendship and AIDS

CONTENTS

Foreword by Bishop Walter F. Sullivan ix

Introduction by Sister Patrice Murphy, S.C., Director, Supportive Care Program, St. Vincent's Hospital, New York, New York xi

ONE.	In the Evening We Will Be Judged by Love...	1
TWO.	Pole Sitting and the Art of Zen.............	15
THREE.	Mike, and the Listener of Last Resort......	29
FOUR.	The Monk Despite All........................	39
FIVE.	Peter, Cary, and the Third Party Lurking.	65
SIX.	The Time Told Awry, the Time Told Right.	123

SEVEN.	Eight Brief Candles.	147
EIGHT.	Oscar; No Story Worth Telling?	161
NINE.	Lost and Found in the Floating Forest.	169
TEN.	Ikon or Idol; and One Who Chose.	185
ELEVEN.	The Dream and the Dreamer.	201
TWELVE.	Epilogue	223

FOREWORD
Walter F. Sullivan
Bishop of Richmond

I list myself among the many admirers of Father Daniel Berrigan, S.J. He witnesses both against the holocaust of nuclearism and the holocaust of abortion. His writings are always poetic and inspirational, his message ever timely and beneficial. The present volume, *Sorrow Built a Bridge: Friendship and AIDS*, is no exception.

Dan has put a human face on AIDS, the malady which has reached epidemic proportions. Over 100,000 persons in the United States have been diagnosed HIV positive with about 58,000 having died from this deadly disease. Dan recounts his own personal journey and ministry with fourteen specific persons for whom "death was given a royal welcome." He does not dwell on the causes of AIDS nor does he pass judgment on its victims doomed to "atrocious suffering".

In moving and descriptive language Dan paints a picture of his own experience of inadequacy and helplessness in the presence of such overwhelming pain. His ministry is mostly one of simple presence, gentle listening coupled with a word of consolation, an invitation to dinner at his own home, and on occasion, a reconciliation with friends and family, with God and church. He vividly describes the experience of the person who suffers the pain of bodily deterioration coupled with the pain of abandonment of friends and loved ones who "walk away."

Father Berrigan gives meaning to his own experience by choosing and reflecting on selected scripture passages. He also connects his encounters with the deaths of those who were once "young and vigorous" with his own peacemaking. In both cases, "dreams turn into nightmares," "old hatreds don new fatigues" and "immunity systems break down both in a person and in a nation."

This book is a special gift to those committed to compassionate care for persons with AIDS. It is not one to be read in a hurried fashion but to be shared in meditative prayer and reflection groups. I, who have occasional contact with persons with AIDS, am grateful to the author for helping me realize that the present crisis is not a divine curse but a true KAIROS, a graced moment when God draws near and challenges each of us to act creatively to make visible the loving God whom "no one has ever seen." (John 1:18.)

INTRODUCTION
Sister Patrice Murphy, S.C.
Director, Supportive Care Program St. Vincent's Hospital, New York, New York

In the 70's a new movement was afoot in the United States. It was a novel idea, at least in the Americas; but actually, it was ages old. It was the hospice movement.

The Oxford English Dictionary defines "hospice" as "a house of rest and entertainment for pilgrims, travellers, or strangers ... for the destitute or sick." Hospices were common as long ago as the Middle Ages—perhaps before, and as just that—places for the weary traveller to rest, become refreshed. The dictionary also reminds us that from the same root (L. *hospes*) are derived hospice, hospitality, host, and hospital.

Sandal Stoddard in her book *The Hospice Movement* comments on this so fittingly:

> Certainly it is a measure ... of the split between mind and heart in the modern consciousness that we have needed a dictionary to help us recover the ancient connection between the objective thing, hospital, and the embracing act, hospitality.

But hospices, thanks to the charism of men and women of various religious orders in medieval Europe, were subtly different from inns where pilgrims could rest and be refreshed on their journeys. The religious hospices came into being because some people, in their journey through life, became old and sick, were poor and even dying, but there were no other people to cherish and console and support those in need. Religious orders, sensitive to such human needs, responded with a love of neighbor rooted in their love of God.

The hospice concept remained largely European until the '70s when, in North America, the work of Dame Cecily Saunders at St. Christopher's Hospice in London and Elizabeth Kübler-Ross in the United States was attracting notice and interest. They were writing and talking about death and dying and the care of the terminally ill and their loved ones. Death, like sex, had been "in the closet." Just as modern society had lost the connection between "hospital" and "hospitality," it also lost a sense of the proper continuity between life and death. The hospice movement emphasizes this continuity.

Dr. Cecily Saunders spoke to this point in a discussion of the modern hospice:

> This is indeed a place of meeting. Physical and spiritual, doing and accepting, giving and receiving, all have to be brought together.... The dying need the community, its help and fellowship.... The community needs the dying to make it think of eternal issues and to make it listen....

So it was with this new look at old truths that thoughtful hospital administrators began to consider the "how" of implementing such concepts—making them live within their institutions and indeed in all of modern health care. They were motivated, too, by a sad awareness which pointed up again the marked difference between "hospital" and "hospitality." Large

Introduction

hospitals, growing daily in size and technical grandeur, dedicated to sorting out and treating all the intricacies of illness—the more interesting, the better—and committed to research and education, these large hospitals were heading in another direction. They were losing sight of those patients who were, perhaps, no longer interesting or challenging, those for whom "nothing more" could be done. Physicians visited such patients less frequently, nurses took a longer time to answer a call bell, visitors were seldom seen, and people whispered about the patient: they could not bear to speak aloud the dreaded word, "dying." What happened to hospitality?

St. Vincent's Hospital and Medical Center of New York was not exempt from such frailties; but the religious leadership in the Medical Center was strong and always alert to and committed to seeking out ways to better serve its patients: the sick, the poor, the dying.

In 1979 St. Vincent's chose a nurse-administrator to develop a hospice program in its center of healing, education, and research. This was a long, arduous, challenging task, but the goals of reverence and comfort—physical, mental, spiritual—for the terminally ill person and his or her loved ones; the goal of providing home care by loving persons; the goal of allowing and even encouraging the dying to continue living with dignity and grace until death—all these goals were well worth the struggles involved.

During the '80s certification and licensing procedures for hospices were drawn up by the government, and these made monetary reimbursement possible for "certified" hospices. (I.e., government tax dollars and statist red tape could now control at least the hospice if not Christian hospitality itself.) Hospices only then became a "viable health-care option" for many modern health care institutions. At St. Vincent's the certification option was explored but rejected. The program, not to mislead either church or state watchdogs and bureaucrats, was named the Supportive Care Program.

Suddenly, in the '80s, the plague-like disease AIDS appeared, killing thousands of talented young people and leaving in its wake terror, grief, and dreadful stigma. Parents turned against children; brothers and sisters were torn apart by conflict; morality and immorality became everyone's area of expertise; and "What will the neighbors think!" became a criterion for behavior even toward one's own. Was there a contribution the Supportive Care Program could make in face of so much suffering? This was no time for cowardice. The message of the Gospel was being lost or abandoned amid tremendous fear and pharisaic righteousness. In a spirit of concern and compassion, the Supportive Care Program became involved in the care of persons with AIDS.

We know that we as caring, competent, knowledgeable, and sensitive practitioners can and have made a difference over the six years of our work with more than 500 persons with AIDS and with their loved ones. The professionals in the program are joined by many valuable and valued, caring volunteers of whom Father Berrigan is one. His help, like that of all who work in the Program, makes hospitality live among the dying. Remembrances of patients similar to the ones in this book are cherished by all who work in the Program even though no one is as beautifully articulate as Father in the remembering.

As the patients daily face debilitating symptoms and profound weakness, aggressive treatments with the possibility of severe side effects, grim prognoses despite valiant efforts to save them, and often, the emotional and spiritual suffering of shame, rejection, prejudice, isolation, and ostracism, the Supportive Care staff intervenes. They try to provide or obtain the best medical and nursing care; they listen to the sadness as they search for hope; they try to discover and respond to the stresses and to the good times (periods of remission) and help pave the way home for any period of time. They minister to the human spirit, trying to mirror the love and compassion of Christ.

Introduction

Because of this Program, hundreds who might have died in isolation, fear, and pain have lived instead as valued individuals; and those left behind in their loss and grief have not had to suffer alone. They too have had the opportunity to experience comfort and healing through the Program's bereavement services.

In sum, the Program strives to blend for each patient just the right proportions of care and caring, nursing and nurturing, medicine and ministry. It serves as a model for other highly motivated persons and groups who wish to make a difference in the lives of terminally ill individuals, particularly those with AIDS. This work is testimony that the Good News, the Gospel is alive and well, and that the cherishing, comforting, compassionate Jesus continues to serve and heal through others.

ONE

IN THE EVENING WE WILL BE JUDGED BY LOVE

It started with a phone call from a nun. There was trouble in her family.

It would seem that the affliction she alluded to should at very least be given a name; especially when, as in this instance, an urgent SOS was being issued.

Eventually the affliction was named by the caller, with fear and trembling. But the illness was by no means dwelt on, as to effect, symptom; above all, cause. Only the terror, the grief.

It was clear once more; the illness in question is more than a disease. It carries a baleful light of the supernatural, it stands oblique and blind and menacing outside medical category. In the mind of the beholder it is mated with deviant conduct, it conjures up dark corners where the unspeakable festers away.

I must add that the voice on the phone held none of this dark coloration of innuendo. It was as though the caller were, in the midst of great suffering, reaching out to a last resort. Fairly straightforwardly: 'My nephew has AIDS. You were on a college faculty with his uncle, a Jesuit, Father So-and-so. Luke has survived for a matter of three years. The latest bout seems final; both cancer and pneumonia. Will you visit him?'

Other talents, other strokes. Our world is a wondrous cornucopia indeed: it contains card sharpers and belly dancers, poets, flamenco guitarists, hang gliders and money-market players—stars of the firmament all, native winners. And then other sorts, drawn, for reasons that utterly escape them (us, me)—drawn to such scenes as AIDS.

These latter will bear scrutiny. They are cursed with a very connoisseurship in such summonses as I describe. They are even found useful there.

To speak shortly, it seems as though the world of pain is their turf; native, never moony or distant. On that planet where humans are born only to go under, they are granted a royal welcome. The world is, alas, densely populated; the planet as terminal ward.

What does the planet look like? Well, for one thing, and here and now—like the ravaged landscape of a single face. Telltale splotches, the color of damp soil. Lazarine, as though the grave spots still clung to the risen. (But here we have the bitter reverse of a miracle, death claiming the young and vigorous.)

. . .

Luke's hospital room was altogether familiar. I could have entered it blindfolded. Nor was it a stranger who languished there; I knew him. Something of a recognition scene, old Walt Whitman or the Latin poet Horace; nothing human foreign to me.

Human indeed. A face pressed by an unseen hand into a new form, new contours of bones, cheek, socket. Death looked out of him, that old taker and giver, mortality and then presto! immortality. I thought, not of death but of Yeats and 'the face I had before the world was made.'

His face was cleared for action, no missing it. Or it was a pro tem face, borrowed. On consignment, was that the phrase?

There would be a day, and not far distant, when the claim fell due.

      . . .

Most days his parents made their way into Manhattan.

They were more or less bewildered, a low voltage panic. In such a world, will someone make sense of it all? Please?

As far as could be judged, there was no God around to tell them the score. There was only brute fact. Reasoning stopped here, solutions there were none. There was only ruin, disaster, blighted hope.

And the priest standing there, what of him?

If truth were told, he was as ignorant as they. An ignorance that was something more than a hiatus in the mind. It was more like a working principle. You might even call it a source of endurance, if not courage.

It went something like this. He knew nothing of the why of God, or the why of AIDS. And he came to the hospital, and stood with the parents and their dying son.

There was a strange kinship here, of ignorance. He knew nothing as they knew nothing; or as near nothing as to make no difference.

The so-called working principle, it went to work. One might even say in a sorry sense, it worked.

In this way: being almost dumb, having little to say, he would not offer false comfort or a quick fix.

Nor would he play God. He knew the only god one could mime in such circumstances was an inferior one, a ventriloquist's doll mouthing someone else's platitudes. So he kept quiet.

Why not? He could offer no formulas to comfort their suffering.

Any more than God did. True God that is, merciless God, the God of Jesus on the cross and 'Why have you forsaken me?' The God of silence, of turning aside, the God of 'not yet,' the God of no comment. The God who bore with extermination camps and torture rooms and the disappeared. The God of this world; a world of contras and wicked judges and drug kingpins and police beatings and abortion abattoirs and electric chairs.

Dare we say: the God who walks this world, who bears with all this, who groans and weeps? who is patient—even with the likes of us?

In any case. The priest's strength (or what passed muster for strength) was a simple act of the will. At least it set the priest free, it relieved his dumb and heavy ignorance, made it bearable. He wanted to be there. To be with this afflicted pair and their son. To go through it all with them. This, he thought, might be the substance of that 'answer' we lust after, and in so lusting, forget to frame the question aright.

A question such as—have You really abandoned us, left us to our sorry resources and sorrier outcomes? Or are You really here, in our midst, helping us find a human way together, two added to two, parents, priest, son? and so doing, come to a peace, a lightness of heart, even laughter now and then?

And summoning a laugh or a cheerful face, can we let the ominous undercurrent flow along, but kept under, where it belongs? I mean that stream, icy and scalding, tears, stalemate, onset of grief, outcries.

These too. But in their time and place.

Meantime, in this place, meeting for the first time, without a word we came to a common resolve. To forbid that current a takeover, determining mood and word, owning us. Like the shadow of a lamprey in a free-running stream. Let it keep its distance.

. . .

A parallel occurs to me, a scene in the gospel. The Lord enters a room where the daughter of the house has died. The family are mourning uncontrollably. And He comes in.

He has no word of comfort. Indeed he speaks sharply, in reproof. As though to ask indignantly, why do you pay unseemly tribute to necessity and nature? As though the Lord of Life could, to any right understanding, arrive 'too late.'

Then it blazes out: 'She is not dead, but sleeping.'

They break out in derision, but he puts them to the door. And proceeds to raise the child from death.

It is that diagnosis of His that clings in the mind. Not dead, but sleeping. Not dying, but going toward life.

. . .

I thought also of a visit a few years back, to Northern Ireland. We arrived in Belfast in the midst of the crisis in Long Kesh prison. We lodged with the families of prisoners, we witnessed their grief and pain; and in those humble homes were treated royally.

And now and again, in this or that pub, we celebrated together.

And this transpired, it must be understood, in the midst of the prisoners' fast, and the death eventually of twelve of them. There we sat with the families and the pub crowd, lifting our ale in salute, singing.

It seemed right to do so. Despite all. Some sixth sense in us went deeper than the brute fact of impending death. Something about surpassing death by celebrating life.

A matter of hope in a bad time. Of hope against a wall, and in that testing, that stalemate, vindicating itself; hope, and no illusion, no base or frivolous substitute.

Those we love (so our hope went) may be taken from us by death. Indeed they will be. But this is hardly the last word; there is more to be said, the Savior has said so. More, he has gone through it all, and come out. He knows whereof he speaks. So we, in face of death, act in the world as though this great thing were true.

The grave is a hole reversed, an empty pocket.

Thus we and the prisoners' families raised our glasses, and sang together, and toasted the dying. Whom we loved and mourned. And more.

This is the strength of that thing we name, and now and again see in its grandeur and strength, 'catholic.'

. . .

Well, there he lay, Luke, master chef, trained in France, lately owner of his own restaurant in Brooklyn.

Now everything was 'lately,' everything on hold. You couldn't miss it in his eyes, in the calm level blur of a voice, bled of emotion. He knew. In his best moments (which were most of them), he was—accepting. Taking what came with a laconic, understated nobility.

He spoke now and then of the good days, the cafe, overseeing waiters, marketing, trying out recipes, pleasing and teasing those finicky New York palates. Mindful, remembering. But not lustful, not nostalgic or resentful. Done with all that.

His hand and foot were swollen and empurpled and twice their normal size. Useless, they lay on pillows like limbs become ikons or relics.

And the parents in the background, greeting the priest. 'Of course we remember you. God knows we heard you preach last New Year's at Saint Francis Xavier.'

Well well.

We had a few memories in common, no great thing. But enough to distill some half-hour into a semblance of reason, the small talk that saves.

I walked with them to the elevator. 'He'll never leave here. Nothing to do but prepare him for a good death.' The mother mourned.

Nothing indeed.

'He's fought so long and so hard.' She looked me longingly in the eye, awaiting something; reassurance. Would he die a 'good catholic?' Would I see to that?

Know it or not, the son was already seeing to that. On his own, with their goodness at his side. Therefore say nothing, for now.

. . .

Against all expectations he went home, swollen limbs and all, the lungs still congested.

I visited his apartment, a small cove in Chelsea. It was snug and neat; in the living room, unusual urban amenities; a fine brick wall and a fireplace.

There he held court, grayfaced, his hair a mere wisp of coarse straw. Death nearing, but on his phiz a smile that turned the heart over. And stuck on his head, visor reversed, the most rakish baseball cap of that or any season.

A fading pro, a dying ballplayer. And no giving up. The season was over, pennants were out, life was a holiday. Hail to the champ!

I brought flowers and a wedge of brie. On the phone, when I asked what I should bring along, he said; 'Of course, brie. I'm not supposed to have it, but what the hell.'

. . .

'Tell me about that restaurant of yours.'
'Well, I came back from France with a bit of money. I wanted to open my own place. So I took out an ad in the *Times*, seeking a partner, and found someone with cash in hand. We rented a storefront in a tough neighborhood. We wanted to do something other than chic, a French and Italian menu, good food at decent prices.

'We took a big chance. And we lost, lasted only a year. I can see now the mistakes we made.'

A faint, lurking regret. That was all.

. . .

A day later, on the phone. 'You know that cheese you brought. I was sick for twenty-four hours afterward.'
'What an ending to a party!'
'Yeah. But didn't we have a good time!'
The news was, he had to go back to hospital. 'I haven't told the folks yet. They'll know soon enough.'
What was it (my heart sinking) this time?
'They want to do an implant in the chest. Something about direct chemotherapy.'
Then; 'Daniel, how did you know when to phone? Your timing's perfect.'
How come?

'Well, I'm alone today, a mixup with the visiting help. I've been trying to reach her, but no go. I worry about her, she has kids.'

I was learning. Down and out is strictly relative. More, down and out is a spiritual matter. It says something about One Body, All of Us.

And relative. Put it way: when life is seen whole and steady, someone else is always downer and outer.

. . .

Some thirty-six years ago I was ordained. Shortly thereafter, I remember preaching on a text of St. John of the Cross; 'In the evening we will be judged by love.'

I think of Luke; and of what a mild and gentle judgment that will be.

My friend will be judged by love. Which is to say, he will not be judged, but embraced.

What draws us to the embrace of love is a courage akin to his. The courage to believe, church and state notwithstanding, the only judgment will be that of love.

. . .

Luke, in his flat New York brogue. In the middle of a discussion on the latest symptomatic horror, he'll suddenly break off, 'Now what about you? What're you up to?'

Courage, he seems to say, no big deal. Thereby indicating by indirection how big a deal it is. Courage sums him up, that sparse, barely ambulatory shadow of a figure, as he makes an old man's way from chair to bed and back again.

. . .

He is much on my mind.

I learn from him. To believe. To say, as seldom before, I believe in the resurrection of the body.

The present state of that body, awful as it is, and appalling as it must be to its person—that body is all the more dazzling and beautiful in its import. For all of that, all taken in account.

His sores are a kind of stunning negative apologia.

The least likely event in all creation is that this frame of his, ruined and rent as it is, and utterly bereft of temporal prospect, should be the subject of apotheosis. That this wasted weakened frame should become a resurrected body, lithe and weightless and free of the awful necessities of mortal flesh?

Nothing less likely, goes the holy illogic. Therefore nothing more true.

. . .

So near removal he is, soon to be thrust out of time and place. He is in a truly spectacular position, a kind of box seat adjacent to eternity. Able from there, from that extraordinary vantage point, to tell what shall shortly be. To tell of resurrection.

Not by dying, certainly (anyone can die; most of us will)—but by living as he does.

. . .

Another visit. He's bound hand and foot to that wheel of grief known as time. In his case, hospital time.

But for his eyes, still lively and watchful, he could already have been consigned to the permanent underground.

. . .

I enter. Someone unidentifiable, masked, is addressing the patient in a high pitched singsong. She is, it appears, the hospital dietitian. Her tones are punishing, she stands at safe distance from the bed and its hypothetical contaminations. Rants on of this and that, and mainly nothing at all.

The scene is hilarious, if one has heart for it. She is revealing as to a little child, certain esoteric information concerning hospital menus. The difference, otherwise unattainable by mortals like him, between pureed and ground food! And all conveyed with deadly seriousness. How to relieve dry fowl 'with a spot of butter or gravy.' And so on.

I listen, my jaw hangs witless. The woman is instructing, apparently without knowing or caring, the quondam chef of a gourmet restaurant of some note.

She departs. We grin like two goblins in the night.

I venture a word of praise for his patience. He receives the tribute equably.

I tell him there is something of his Jesuit uncle about him; I remember a modest man of scholarly achievement, and a splendid teacher.

'Too bad I never got to know him well, he was always the scholar and I had no talent in that direction.'

. . .

I returned one day, he was sleeping. I sat within range of his eyes. His poor sunken eyes opened and slowly focused. I was wearing a white shirt, Indian fashion, against the heat of the season.

'Good God,' he quipped hoarsely. 'That beautiful shirt! I thought for a moment we'd both made it.'

. . .

I was not to see him again. Within days he was in better hands than ours. Faith, though blind with tears, assures us it is so.

His mother wrote, 'Luke was the peacemaker in our family. He had great courage and a wonderful sense of humor. . . . Just in the last weeks of his life, when he and I had a quiet moment alone, he took my hand in his and said, "I know I'm not leaving the hospital, but I've accepted it. It's all right, but I'm concerned for you and Dad. Please don't grieve for me."'

He meant the request with all his rugged failing heart. And he knew it could not be honored.

'We grieve for him,' his mother continued, 'but we know that he is with the Lord and at peace and freed from his terrible suffering.'

TWO

POLE SITTING AND THE ART OF ZEN

Ambrose is twenty-nine, a slight gamin figure. He sits disconsolate as I enter. Greeting me, he summons from some depth where courage takes its source, a wan smile.

Ambrose is a homophobe's delight. If the elements of a merciless unloving caricature were assembled in one frame, Ambrose would qualify. He is skinny and birdlike, excessively given to pursing of lips and bobbing of head. His gestures are airy and inconclusive, his frame shrunken by long wasting.

Nothing of a cynical and hateful world, no malevolence, dread, fear, or the like could possibly vanquish the innocence and sweetness of the man. How easily stereotypes dissolve!

I hold out a hand, announce myself as 'a friend of Sister Pat; she asked me to stop by.'

No hand of Ambrose meets mine. Only that ghost of a smile, and a merest emanation of a voice, faint as though also issuing from a ghost.

How nice of you, and of Sister.

His eyes remain fixed and open, gazing into the distance.

Ambrose is nearly blind. His affliction, on the crosshatching of unpredictables called AIDS, was like no other I had encountered. Meningitis.

He is so lonely. Friends and family come by, but the days are long, his weakness extreme. There is music, and around the holiday season, fanciful creations of flowers, leaves, ribbons, appear. They mitigate the scene, but given his plight, the favor is done more for visitors than for him.

He says, 'I see the shadows of beautiful things and faces, but that is all.'

He had been prosperous, and for so young a person, had won a certain fame as an interior decorator. Two rather glitzy magazines reposed on the window sill. He invited me, after my second visit, to peruse them; 'Some work I've done,' and then a long sigh; 'but that's all over now.'

Several pages in each issue were devoted to Ambrose, his tastes and proclivities, as these had transformed two wealthy lairs into very caves of Aladdin; an urban apartment and a country home.

. . .

Another visit; and another visitor has preceded me. His uncle, a loquacious billboard of a man, a former mailman from Queens, I am told. Informed of my name, he took to pronouncing it repeatedly. 'Berrigan, Berrigan,' musingly. 'Could it be? One of the famous brothers?'

Ambrose perked up, head to one side. 'Berrigans? What brothers? Who are they?'

'Who are they? My boy, where have you been all your life? Why, they. . . . '

It was funny and distressing, both. Ambrose's sightless eyes widened, his face grew animated, he was like a child in a nursery hearing for the first time, 'Once upon a time. . . . '

I knew it, here comes the past again, God help us; here comes trouble.

Ambrose, dear Ambrose, you're not the only one bombarded by stereotypes. Once more the media have 'done their job';

reaching even into this innocent room of yours. Homophobes? Please, the media are omniphobes.

Now what to do? How undo, or at least limit, the harm?

How I longed for the pre-avuncular days of innocence, Ambrose and I free to be ourselves, I a mere friend entering his room from time to time, no big deal.

I am fingered by Queensboro savvy. Henceforth, if the past held a clue to the future, I am to be known only as a 'political priest,' a peculiar type. Someone about whose faith or hope or church connection little is known, but much can be surmised. Someone whom the media have tainted with a faintly noisome smell—of the suspect, the notorious.

From now on, Ambrose would receive me differently.

How could I offer him the simple and holy courtesies available to my kind, a blessing, a prayer for healing? Would he henceforth dread my coming, or merely tolerate it, sensing a hidden agenda somewhere, fearing the mythic blast of a revolutionary bullhorn?

How I cursed the media in my heart, consigned them one and all to the blackest nether regions. Those liars and princes of lies, those dealers in horror and figment, casting their false images on walls and souls. Never mediating, always impeding, making sport and mockery of truth.

How difficult to stand before the children, the ill, the Ambrose kind—and be oneself! and be received as oneself.

If he was victimized, I reflected, so was I. If America 'solved' his existence by consigning him to the high culture of country estates and urban penthouses, it was also skilled in ways of shunting aside the likes of me.

I was at the mercy of folly and appetite and the marked money of the culture. My truth was tossed into this lethal mix, all but lost there; the truth of my life.

· · ·

It may be that I make too much of a slight incident, a slight encounter with a dying child of the culture.

The culture, I knew, had destroyed Ambrose; and wished me destroyed as well. If it could but make of me in fact what it purported at large, to make of me.

If it could blind me—to who I was, to my vocation to truth. And with the poison of celebrity (or the obliterating poison of nonentity inflating—it was all the same) could impose another form on my soul. The form it chose from the cultural bestiary: a goat perhaps, or a monkey, or a swine.

Our fight was strangely the same, Ambrose's and mine. He must fight to stay alive, or give it all up. And so, in a parallel way that would bear much pondering, must I.

· · ·

I came back each week; Ambrose seemed to gain confidence. It was possible, after a few more occasions, simply to talk, one to one; less and less smog was in the air. And at the end of our visit, I could lay a hand on his head and pronounce a blessing, a plea for healing. Thus we overcame.

· · ·

He returned home, the doctors having reamed and wrung him and done their worst best. He would have no more of it, he swore. I visited him in his dark chic cave in mid-Manhattan. He was content to see the weeks or months through, at home. No more hospital. He died peacefully three months later.

· · ·

Certain immunity systems long ago broke down, in the nation; even in the nation in the making. Robert Lifton would say: We transgressed a taboo. The Indian wars were the original sin. They were won, the story goes. What had been a taboo (at least among certain religious groupings, Mennonites, Quakers) was violated. A rule was imposed, a clue to an imperial future. If you can't include them, if they refuse for some fool reason to join the winners, wipe 'em out.

. . .

In my tradition, an immunity system exists from the beginning. God is irremediably on the side of life, creates life from inert dust, cherishes life, finally sends an embassy of life, a very Son. A true blood brother. His ethic is one with his life and death, his initiatives and commands issue from the deepest springs of grace; love your enemies, do good to those who lay violent hands on you. Thus you become godlike.

. . .

Jesus gained immunity from death by passing through death, rather than inflicting it. The choice held firm, though the chips were falling, and the choices dire. It was a hard irony, a great scandal, a stone in the path. It impeded the good life, natural reason was slowed, as were prudence and good sense and the purported sanity of the great and powerful. A scandal was born—a scandal among Christians, adept as we grew in the above-mentioned ploys and dodges of the mind.

Thus our irony, the irony of immunity through submission, has its source in the God who formulated it. Jesus, the Original Immune One, God of Life, giver of life, stumbled and fell—

over the paradox, one might say, the scandal, the cross. And this, even as, to the world's satisfaction, the paradox stood firm. The God of life would be put to death. For the world was unattuned to Life; as message, as truth, as consonant music. It was attuned to death—to the dealing and undergoing, the method and madness, dissonance and muffled drumbeat, Diplock and deception. The power that corrupts was infinitely preferable to the powerlessness that enhances.

Words bumble about, making much ado over a simple and beautiful (one would even dare say a self-evident) thing.

. . .

Death is a brute fact, but sin is a drama, a moral and tragic movement, within a soul, within a social body. Assaulting the life of the Immune One, the sin (rampageous power, ego, the military and its sycophant courts and jails) despite its dead weight, is drawn toward a further event, a milestone, an outcome. And over this victorious progression of grace and the outcry of life, sin exerts less and less command; eventually death meets its opposite and vanquisher. Which we name now and again, in moments relatively unswamped by the world, resurrection.

I have this sense, which is so difficult to express, except perhaps in signs; faces, cries, bread and wine, the sweet water of the world cupped in a hand. Art even (and within limits).

. . .

As I set down these notes, a new judicial gavel thumps down on me and my friends. The public breakdown leaves social systems in shambles. We see this again and again as we sit in the school of that merciless teacher named experience.

I think of a dying 'system of justice.' What does it look like, in its last days?

We go into court as we might visit a ward of a mental hospital. Someone is ill, perhaps beyond healing; there are vivid overmastering illusions, language contrary to fact, bizarre ignorance, glacial self confidence.

The 'visitors' are still on their feet, responsible, in command of their powers. They are quite capable, if allowed, of explaining their conduct, connecting it with a sane and civilized tradition. They insist on a hearing, not for themselves merely. For the children, the unborn, the gentle harboring earth. They are in good health. And like all so gifted, they offer health to others.

Alas, the court is something more terrible even than our metaphor suggests; it is weighted with a stale mortuary air. An unaccountable ritual is in progress, its protocol both turgid and rigid. Here, surely, one pales in the imminent presence of death. Something has broken down; the dead are celebrating death.

. . .

It has been said in other ways, and better. It merits saying once more; the way of Jesus and the way of the Bomb are absolutely, metaphysically incompatible. The statement might seem, were the world sane and the church Christ-like, impossibly redundant. Because neither is either, the statement becomes, though otiose to some, a necessary drumbeat.

. . .

Here goes with another metaphor.

America has learned to make of the ancient teaching called transmigration of souls, a useful cultural tool. I mean something like this: practically everyone in America, at one time or another, has transmigrated, soul and body, family and job, goods and chattels, skills, prejudices, political leanings, ancestry and progeny, from somewhere to somewhere else. Geographically, geopolitically, religiously, the beat goes on; a diverse, at times perverse, cacophony. It sounds loud in marriage, friendship, responsibility toward one's community at large, one's own children.

Now and then, one grants reluctant kudos to all this, a method in madness—maybe out of bewilderment, or a sense that almost anything capable of shedding light on our darkness ought to be welcomed.

Some, in despair of domesticated versions of religious faith, look abroad in longing. Oh for the whirling dervishes, another exotic time and place! If only one could learn the steps, a new dance! This wild furor of monads, seemingly without rhyme or reason—could it not discover for us whether life has meaning at all, where, if anywhere, our leaps and feints might land us?

The foregoing occurred to me, more exactly in regard to my friends, the ill. All were formerly in good health and spirits. And all, alas, are presently neither, a transmigration of fates, indeed; and sorrowful beyond telling.

The fates push hard, and further. There are terrifying transitions, molds broken and mended (or broken and discarded). The ill describe themselves; formerly religious (or irreligious), formerly married, formerly 'sexually active,' and often formerly skilled and well paid, well heeled, well loved. So much formerly!

This is what dying means, I thought; the drama of 'formerly' yielding, with infinite pain and loss, to the drama of—what? Emptyhandedness, the broken vessel; where one is, and shortly will not be; what one is, and shortly will not be.

And then, a strange meantime! One lives there, at the mercy (or mercilessness) of others. Career blasted, income as well. Little remains under the sway of choice, friends and family desert ship. The church likely as not an ambiguous hoverer, judge, punisher, only now and again healer or savior.

And what remains? Faith, perhaps. Deepened, in spite of the worst.

Or destroyed by the Destroyer, the angel whose breath is impure darkness.

. . .

Among the ill are husbands and fathers; only rarely a wife or mother. In at least one instance, the wife no longer wants sight of the former spouse; neither do the children. We must find a place for him. With AIDS added to the woman's burden, raising the children alone, who wants a walking Job on the scene? And who knows if AIDS, close up, might even infect the children?

. . .

Back to St. Vincent's. I cannot forget my friend, Ambrose. Images of him, memories recur. Ambrose. 'Something childlike about him,' says Sister Patrice.

Indeed. He lies there, his hair on end like a straw thatch, weak, weak. And anon, a spasm seizes him, and he begins to shake uncontrollably. I run for the nurse. She rushes in. He pops the Tylenol (ugh), and relief comes.

. . .

Then he's at home again, coping, though blind by meningitis. He has crawled through the very knothole of Job, a passage months long; dragging his arse with only minor contusions, through and through, to the other side.

'I'm a stark realist,' this diminutive number declares in his reedy voice, 'even though my parents aren't.' And how right he is, at least in his description of his own adamant will—to live, even to recover his health, grateful as he is for the least sign of comeback.

He reminds me of a circus act on one of those immensely tall steel poles. The performers shinny up, nimble and nonchalant, cavorting as they climb. The steel bends and sways, like the most fragile of reeds. Eventually one of the performers perches topmast on each pole, quite as though born to such unlikely heights.

Now the pole climbers become pole sitters; they sway about like ripe fruit in a wind, greet their peers, just like the 'fire folk sitting in the air' of the Hopkins poem. They even exchange perches nonchalantly, perform any number of unlikely jumps and pirouettes across the void.

My steely little friend! He too has climbed, he has earned his unsteady perch in the world.

. . .

'I couldn't face the hospital again. I find the very thought mentally disturbing. So we're praying nothing comes up to force me to return. . . . '

Such bravery awakens image after image.

He resembles the famous Unkle Geedunk in the movies, purblind, knocking into everything; at the same time, absolutely unfazed, wildly combating the pterodactyls of the night as they flap and caw about his ears.

Or in my mind the little gent sits in a thimble of a lifeboat, the epitome of a survivor. There he abides, utterly blind as to direction, without cares. My image by no means multiplies his actual woes. He's stripped of every instrument of human surcease. Shark meat. No succor in sight. Rocking and drifting, barely this side of disaster and death.

His mood is pure zen.

No one is in sight, neither help nor intervention, no deity of deep nor sky to lend a hand. Nevertheless, begone cynicism, begone despair! He is innocent of worry as is the deep or the faultless sky above. His soul is a mirror of each of these; this is his triumph, his lucid humanity. His hope walks the waters, the immense contrary element. Or he takes wings, he is a child of the ether.

Ready for heaven, brother to me.

It is unimportant that he know any of the foregoing.

It is important only that he be . . . as he is. It is important for me to know his longitude and latitude, so to speak; since it is through his and his like that I take the soundings of my existence. Where I am. Somewhere. Near him.

. . .

This strange attempt to account for times both malfeasant and beneficent continues.

I had hardly thought, when I started this hospice work, that the thing would move so close, like a mysterious body sliding through a window at midnight, all menace, a greater darkness in the darkness. One awakens in a stupor; who is this interloper? I thought death came by day, when I was in control of the house; never got beyond the door, was dealt with, bargained with, dismissed there. . . .

But this one is a break-in, stakes out his turf. I can turn angry all I want, or panic. Or I can call the police.

He knows it; they won't come anyway.

THREE

MIKE AND THE LISTENER OF LAST RESORT

Resumé, as conveyed on a first visit.

An actor and teacher of acting. Quaker, sometime Methodist. Park Avenue address. Presently between stages in hospital. Home, breathing free; for awhile.

In appearance and demeanor, childlike, vulnerable—an achievement, no artifact as I've come to know.

Yes, came the message, he would be delighted to meet me. And that same day, if convenient. He must first, in early afternoon, be taken to Central Park by a nurse for a wheelchair outing.

He gave a somber account of those two hours. 'I suppose an actor is hyper about such things. But it's terrible, the way people stare at me.'

'Why would they stare at you?'

'It has something to do with my being young, and the fact that I'm chair-bound. You can almost read it in their eyes, I wonder if he's. . . . '

I ventured it was important to ignore such bad manners. He supposed so, but oh, it was hard. . . .

. . .

His dwelling was an 'air shaft condo'; it looked out on a blank courtyard; an apartment you once could buy for a song, now its price would strip an entire forest of its singing birds. A formidable art piece centered the living room: a contraption, some eight feet by four feet, composed of wires, colored plastic inserts, and hidden lighting. It glimmered away, off, on, in the gentle spring twilight like the eye of a vigiling daemon.

He began easily, a long monologue of grief, relieved now and again by a reflective smile.

So simple a thing was transpiring; we were becoming friends.

'Friendship? In "normal" times, times so distant, so plain unimaginable, as to tick away only in folk tales—at such times it flowered of itself, was governed by its own laws.

'You encountered someone in the course of school or work or play, you drifted closer, the chemistry worked well. Time together went easy, there was bonding, talk, meals, excursions, vacations. The satisfactions of good work, of making it professionally.

'Thus one friend emerges out of the pack.

'And now a special outcome is invoked. Two settle in. The friends have become lovers, they pledge fidelity. The vows, if the two are lucky, hold. The analogy is a good marriage.'

. . .

Then, to summon events that of recent years have become notorious, disaster strikes.

A faint rumble at first, unease, 'symptoms.' Friends, as one well knows, have been stricken and died. The brutal question insinuates itself like a demon at the door: Can this terror strike me also?

The demon is presently, by some means or other, settled in the parlor, a companionable horror. He's a master of innuendo.

Rumors swirl around him, gather force like a tornado. (But tornados always hit the next town.)

The twister spins about, and dives. From the sky a smoky finger veers about mindlessly, then points. It's like a war poster, benevolent and malevolent at once; Uncle wants you.

Disbelief, panic, the world is post-tornado, a landscape of disaster.

. . .

Life was once a dance. But the dance, so beautifully, impeccably choreographed, is scattered, broken up.

I'm reminded of an old movie, title long forgotten. In one elaborate scene a splendid ball is in progress, a Vienna extravaganza whose mounting was so dear to Hollywood in the Forties. The cotillion moves with precision, the military officers and their ladies preen and bow and whirl, resplendently garbed.

It is the witching hour; the women form (if one may be inelegant among the Brummells) a kind of backup coterie of admiration and ornament and perfumed enticement. Male and female God made them; for this.

And they shine beyond measure. The women are the larger adornment, complement and foil of the military cockatoos. Together they exude the sexuality of violence like a spoor; coercive, intoxicating.

Male and female God made them, like figures circling a music box God made them, tinkling away, telling the time—and all wrong.

How read the time aright? We shall shortly be told. It is the time of . . . disaster.

Cannons boom. The grand city, comatose, feverish, is under assault.

Of a sudden, uproarious winds, havoc seize upon the splendid palace. The casements are blown open, the portieres lift wildly in the air. And the dance breaks up in chaos and wailing and distemper. O what, O who, O whence?

The music box goes mad; the figures fall apart one from another, tumble to ground, broken dolls.

. . .

In sum. We have done with light opera and minuet and smiles of a summer night. We are thrown back bodily in time; Greek ghosts walk abroad in the windblown hall. The stage darkens, the tale unfolds; it is older than the living, its outcome lays all bare—the perfidy and nobility, the chafing of spirit upon spirit, the greed and dandyism and blindness, that hodgepodge of the human; everything the dance celebrated, concealed, knew and did not know.

How the living stand transfixed among the dead. A chorus intones it, the long-lost, long-despised truth; mortality, reality. You were blind, ignorant as the unborn. But no longer. Your healing may commence.

. . .

I think of the larger circle also; of those hierophants once celebrating so strenuously the good life, those buddies of Fire Island and the Hamptons and the gay bars. What of them, where are they, when trouble intrudes so monstrously?

Many of them stand firm, undertake the passage at the side of those they love. This is a great hope that touches on friendship everywhere; friends sustaining, refusing to give up, and so diffusing the terror.

Indeed fidelity begins here; with the capability of bearing disaster. A disaster that touches more than the ill, since all gays are threatened with a like bleak outcome.

The quality of friendship; standing firm under duress. This, it seems to me, is a summons to all the living.

. . .

And some walk away. We stand at a crossroads; the ancient Greeks called it 'Krisis.'

And I come to another form of an old game; in my life too, many have walked away, others have stood with me. Indeed my life continues in this rhythm; rejection, embrace.

And what strikes far more deeply than the pain of loss is the gain. The sheer surprise, the gift, imaginative, unexpected, of those who walk with me.

Who could have dreamed such a blessing? More to the point, who could have deserved it?

. . .

Another visit to my afflicted friend. I was welcome, he assured me, though of late he had undergone bad days.

I brought roses along, and a book.

I found him lethargic; still, it was clear his vocal capacities were undiminished. He lay there on the couch exhausted, his tormented swollen legs eased on pillows. And talked and talked.

I have a feeling at times that I am appointed 'listener of last resort'; the one who is near enough, and distant enough to be trusted with matters generally held secret. Invariably, the talk centers on memory and religious faith.

'It was terrible, the religion they foisted on us,' he mourned. 'No end of threats, punishments, hellfire. I took the full brunt. Years and years before I shook it off. I went away to college, and I found the strength to say: enough.'

'Then I came on the Quakers, a joy to this day. Now I can worship a God of mercy, in my own way; maybe this is how we all end, if we're lucky.'

. . .

I spoke of the weekend just past, a retreat I had taken part in. Of a ninety-year-old artist, who came upon our group and invited herself in 'just to see what's going on here.' How we welcomed her, entranced with her feisty spirit.

She responded with sturdy alacrity; could she show us her art? Indeed she could. The drawings were hauled in and placed about the walls. Then, standing before each in turn, she proceeded to deliver an extempore monologue. 'You see this is how I see the world, which is no different perhaps than the way you see it. Maybe, though, I linger a bit longer over this or that?'

Linger she did, for the entire weekend.

. . .

I had succeeded in shifting his attention. Perhaps he could infer something; how others survived, and with what style. He was soberly attentive.

. . .

He is ill-tempered with the nurses, who, according to him, tend toward the overbearing. 'At times the pain is so overwhelming, I just want to pass the day in bed, reviving from a sleepless night. But they won't allow it,' he wailed. 'I must be forever up and doing things. Doing what?'

It seemed to me important that at least now and then he be allowed to run his own show; and said so.

I found it disturbing, too, that his pain went unrelieved. Told of the Brompton Cocktail, a liquid mix of drugs that could be taken at need. Why was not something similar available to him? I promised to consult the nurse.

. . .

He sees his situation so clearsightedly! No sweet talk, no beating about the bush.

And the eternal plaint of stricken youth. 'So many plans I had, so much undone. And now this. Who would have thought. . . . ?'

I know now what 'tongue tied' means. His revelations, straight from a broken heart, bind the tongue to silence.

. . .

I produced, on departing, another gift, a book. With a little prelude. 'These are stories of those I love. To help you know me better.'

He was politely grateful. And I held his hand, told him he was in my heart, that his friends would see him through. He listened, nearly in tears. And so we parted.

But not for long.

. . .

I walked home through the park, absorbing it all. Knowing there is no getting used to their dying, to the plain injustice of it.

Unfair, unfair; if the world were all, and talent thus thwarted and youth brought to naught.

And yet, and yet. The world is by no means all.

My friend too knows this, in the very pit of the dark night . . . of unknowing.

FOUR

THE MONK
DESPITE ALL

Hard to imagine, harder to foresee, the change that comes toward the end.

Thus; in a few short days Aley was literally transformed. He went from volubility, exuberance, a rollicking eye upon the world, into a wide-eyed, childlike silence.

Other voices were murmuring at his inner ear. He lay there, only half turned to us, the remnant of a smile on his face; as one whose attention is drawn powerfully elsewhere.

In the hospital I made bold to ask him one day (a visit when I came on him without others in attendance) what was the state of his spirits? He said, unaccustomedly laconic; 'Good; you know they bring me communion each day here.'

I was thus invited to fill in the interstices, and draw my own conclusions.

And the end can be briefly recounted. He was discharged from hospital. I awaited a phone call, yielding up information; the whereabouts of his digs, his phone number. Alas, another geography beyond all numbers and neighborhoods was soon to be his.

The following Sunday morning he was found dead. His friend the nun had gone to Chelsea, alarmed that nothing had been heard of him for several days. The phone was off the hook.

Had he known something unknown to us? Sensing death, did he choose to face it alone? If so, the act was hardly in character. But there was that sea change to be taken in account, a new found silence, a withdrawal into his cocoon. He died as he lived; monkishly.

. . .

There is no rationing of grief these days, it comes in great doses, like a bolus that would clog the throat of a pachyderm. That same Sunday morning, a call from England informed me of the suicide of a young friend and namesake.

Aley is gone, so is Daniel. Both young, each flung out of natural course and orbit. Aley, so in love with life. But zest failed him as the day went under; silence became his mood and recourse. I walked my rooms, dumfounded and numb. And after a time, my soul counseled me; Aley was spared the long travail; despite all, he was one of the lucky ones.

Of the younger Daniel, what to say? He could not bear 'the world, the way it goes.' Of his madness, his repeated attempts to destroy himself, and especially of the source of his chaos within, I had ample sympathy; perhaps more than was entirely healthy.

His madness was a kind of hyper sanity. His judgment was correct. The world he could not bear has gone mad in its main parts. To judge such a world sane and sound, to make peace with its crimes, is but another form of the self-destruction which the times both induce and restrict.

Given the times, the crimes, it is not to be wondered at that madness erupts in this or that soul (invariably the most sensitive, the least able to 'make do,' to accept folly as virtue, to join the herd). No wonder that the knife is drawn against one's own veins, and the blood let. The act is a bitter commentary, a counter, a last resort. Were the world not blind, it would know that in such an outcome, the hand was raised in judgment against itself.

I must rein in my grief, lest it pull me under.

. . .

We held a memorial Mass for Aley. Since the troubles began between the local church and the gays, such events are transferred to a dingy hall on West 13th Street. I thought as I entered; here we have the equivalent of a Southern black church, flimsy, slapped up, apt for torching—as so often happened in the Sixties; and is presently happening in gay communities as well.

Mass was celebrated by a little slick-haired priest, evidently a regular minister to the outcasts. Prior to the worship he sought me out, introducing himself as being 'in good standing.' I wondered at the curious credential.

It was the Mass of the first Sunday in Lent. The Gospel is from Matthew, and recounts the triple temptation of Jesus in the desert. The priest improved the occasion by a sermon of sorts, presenting himself as a 'mental health worker,' surely another elusive coinage. He proceeded to expatiate on the need to 'improve oneself as a Lenten exercise.

The arcane construct known to him as 'Mental Health' seemed at issue. I sat there woodenly, cheated, reflecting that I might have been attending a lecture on the theory of bootstraps and the self-made man (sic), rather than a Catholic eucharist. But perhaps the thought was evidence of the low estate of my Mental Health.

Poor Aley. His diminutive frame had broken under the bludgeoning of life; but at least he had been spared this dimwitted travesty.

Someone announced prior to the Mass that after communion, we would be free to utter our memories, stories, thoughts of Aley.

I joined the line for communion. The nun who had stood by Aley through the awful months and welcomed him into her home held the chalice. I whispered a thank you to her eyes and fled the scene.

. . .

In this work you make friends—but it is all out of due course and process. There is no common leaf mold of memories to prod alive, to call up for comfort or sweetness. You and your ill friend find yourselves in one dark pocket of circumstances. And you have no past to speak of; no lazy summer days at the beach, no wandering aimless in the streets of the city, no whims engaged or humming in tune. Not once did you two sit leisurely to a meal in the way of friends, when the moon comes up and time is of less account than the man in the moon.

There is nothing of this sweet aimlessness, this world and time enough, which is the indelible mark of friendship and its very civility. No freebootery or spendthrifting, no letting things be for growth of decline—or even for falling out, which haply occurs rarely and for a time only.

No. In this matter, this work with the ill, there is something other than all this; friendship, let us name it, but with a sea change. An errand is in mind, what the Christians would call, I suppose, a 'mission.' Two have been aimed straight at one another, like arrowheads in a contest. There is a willed occasion, there are rules; above all there is urgency. Time has grown tyrannical; he taps the clock face and glares.

The arrangement, the coming together (alas for a few months, or if lucky for a deuce of years)—it is like a mockup of providence. One is free, but had best be ready for a supernal finger that points you and him toward one another; a gesture, could one see the face that directs it, both wan and implicitly tragic.

Friendship indeed; instant, on demand? Rare, let it be said, at least in my life, where friends commonly grew up together, twin branches from a root, over long savannas of time.

'Remember how we first met?' One is hard put to recall. It is like inquiring of a tree of a century, when a first ring of growth started its round.

Now the clocks are gone crazy, the signposts are all awry.

It is something like trying to introduce a noon sun to a setting sun; in a sense, the one is counterpart of the other, parts, images of an identical burning self.

But wait! a few hours will show the truth; the white-hot face is one with the panoplied headdress, the painted face going under. They are one and the same. Give them time (give yourself time!).

. . .

I was in the quandary of one who can tell his own time right, or so it was said. I could also, as they say, take my sweet time; it was high noon. And yet I must meet on the moment, someone made of very sunset. Someone going under.

It could be argued, and was, that the sight of sunset at noon ought to be instructive; for in a way both ghastly and true, my true time was being tolled for me; even though strangely out of kilter, and read by other eyes than mine.

Someone dying, and I not dying. Not as yet. Though of a certainty, my fate is one with his. Meantime, conceivably, my health might prove of benefit, a kind of collateral loan. We would talk of this, or not, he was welcome (briefly) to stand

. . .

We call life so; formless, colorless. We know it is not true. Nothing on earth is without form or color, unless it be angelic or demonic or of the Uncreated Spirit. Least of all are we without color or form, bodily as we go about, bumping and groping and making our way as best we can, with as little harm (indeed, we pray, with a measure of succor) as may be possible.

. . .

So I arrive, interruptively in a manner of speaking, at the door of another. He has been informed of me, as I of him, at least in general terms. Like two peaceable dogs, we will sniff one another out, trot along side by side for awhile. If this is to happen.

Let me put the matter, as I pause with lifted hand to knock this door to attention, in a puzzle, first posed by Isak Dinesen.

It goes like this. Each of us, he on one side of the portal, I on the other, each of us holds the key to a locked box in possession of the other.

. . .

A little ferret of a man, Venezuelan. Eyes bright as the newborn. You would not have guessed, from his bearing, his broad smile, the consonants that softened to a sweetness on his tongue—would not have guessed the trouble that was on him.

He was dwelling for a time in the back bedroom of a brownstone in my neighborhood. Nowhere else to go, he was given living space by a compassionate nun.

His story would wring the heart of a saber-toothed tiger.

Some time before, when his condition was first diagnosed, he had been evicted. Not from an apartment or house, be it known, but from a monastery.

Then, returning to New York, he was welcomed and granted a haven. Two reactions to this plight; almost, one thought, two brands of Christianity.

He was still bearing the wounds of the monks' decision that put him out the door.

Still, I found him cheerful, self contained, voluble.

. ! .

I ring the outside bell, he appears at the second-story window, throws a key out, I catch it (or miss and retrieve), open the outer door and climb the rickety stairs; it's a New York ritual. He's waiting at the apartment door. There's a smile of welcome; I'm to learn how rarely the smile fails him.

There's also a cat in residence, a pair of superlunary orbs gleam through the dusky air, taking my measure. Shades are drawn against the heat. The cat sniffs about my legs, backs away, then takes off; I'm no big deal.

Aley's much given to Latino amplitude of speech; a monologic man. Delightful. His face positively goes alight when he catches sight of me.

We settle in for talk. Talk, as it develops, is his mainstay, his main mast riding the storm, his candle lit against the darkness. Watch him, he will sweet talk demon death into . . . what? A reprieve at least.

Those black eyes of his positively dance in his head, cavort like jumping beans. Under his hands the tepid, slovenly air of July grows lively, he stirs it to a froth, a witch's wondrous brew.

Or he's like a Neapolitan pizza wizard, operatically juggling a doughy substance into shape.

He gives shape to things. Vigorously he expatiates, warming to his subject; friendship, the monastery, his travels.

He misses greatly the discipline and community that 'kept me going, kept me on the ball.' Being on his own now, he's less apt to 'do things for myself, including prayer.'

An impression grows that first time, of a lonely man, out of orbit, doing his best. He longs mightily for his own place; feels not only constrained to one room, but imposing on the goodness of another.

. . .

Weeks go by, I'm to leave town for a teaching stint. And a thought strikes me. Why not invite Aley to live in my place while I'm away? I make the suggestion, he demurs. 'But it'd only be worse afterward, having to come back here again.'

'Well, think it over, talk it over. Call the two weeks a vacation. Why waste time on regrets? A good time is a good time.'

Thus my persuasion.

I left town, he moved in.

It was the neatest ploy in the history of the Big Apple. He watered the plants, read, enjoyed television, cooked for himself; led the gentlest monastic life imaginable. On my return I found everything shining, and a note of thanks.

. . .

In his digs, the cat rules the roost. Adroit as a mountain goat, it climbs about, leaps into the unlikeliest places, wreaks a mindless mild havoc, generally by inadvertence. And afterward, when a vase has fallen or books tumbled to the floor, it looks about with the glance of a guilty child awaiting consequence. Of which there is, generally speaking, none, or only the lightest exasperated pursing of lips and a 'scat!'

Then it ambles off with a twitch of the shoulder, until the next foray.

The feline's culinary requirements seem, to a rather jaundiced eye, somewhat excessive. The sight of ordinary cat food turns up its patrician nose. Feeding time approaching, there must take place vast and complex mixings and cullings and measurings from various cans and jars, to fortify the animal and set its juices flowing. When it finally settles in to the business of eating, the dish is approached with an air of persnickety condescension; a favor is being conceded to mortals.

. . .

As in most of these ventures, we arrive at a rhythm of sorts.

When Aley is up to it, we venture on Broadway and make our way to a coffee shop nearby. He orders tea, I a cappucino.

I ask about his time in the monastery. As on practically any subject under the sun, he's ready to roll.

Was he happy there, was it working for him?

Oh yes, by all means. In time, they offered him the status of 'postulant,' which meant that he was on his way; not yet a monk by any means, not even a novice. Still, he had a status of sorts; he wore a robe that distinguished him from visitors, he was assigned to work in the kitchen, he attended services in the chapel and took his meals with the community. In short, he had approached the gate, was admitted and assigned a place—just inside the door.

Then what?

'Well,' his lively eyes darkened, 'I got sick, that's all. The doctors took a long time coming on what was wrong, I guess they didn't expect AIDS in the cloister. But there it was.'

He lifted his shoulders, raised his hands.

'The news got to the Father Abbot, of course. He was ver' kind, but he had to esplain the canon law to me. Since I was not a monk under vow, there was no way they could agree to keep me in the monastery. I mus go.'

From then on, the tale seemed like a page out of a medieval chronicle, laced with such implausibilities as are still said to exist in such places.

To wit. 'I ask the Father Abbot if I can speak to the community, tell them about my illness, why I am leaving. He say no, he himself would speak to them, after I depart.

'Immediately they take me out of the kitchen. Bango like that! There seem to be such ignorance about this illness, he's afraid someone will say, Why oh why did you let him cook our food?'

'So I leave. I sneak out while the community is in chapel. That way, the Father Abbot says, is best. He can tell them afterward.'

It wrings the heart dry. Can it be imagined, such things still transpire on this planet? In this church?

.   .   .

Let us, even as the realists, canonists, rigorists cavil, wax unreal.

Let us imagine Father Abbot taking counsel with himself, on occasion of the Bad News Revealed.

'On the one hand,' he reflects, 'and beyond any doubt, there is to be taken in account, the law. A good thing perhaps, undoubtedly formulated by sound Christian minds.

'But let us look more closely at the matter before us. The matter of this little would-be monk. In all details relevant to his sojourn among us, he has given satisfaction. He is devoted to his work, cheerful of mien, recollected in spirit. Most suggestive of all, he is well loved among the brethren.

'As to his illness and its possible ramification, it must be concluded, and plainly stated to the community, that he seems quite capable of living a celibate life. And as far as anyone knows (as far as is known, let it be added, about any member of the community) this postulant has so lived.

'The law is clear in the matter, alas. And this little brother of ours, Aley, is ill. By every indication, ill unto death. And what is to be done?'

Not easy. The law is clear, as always; the application damnably unclear.

As usual.

'He is our brother; the numb.' The matter of the Great Command. The gospel is clear too; and this clarity, issuing from the mind and heart of the Savior, then dawning on us (dogging us) is no consolation at all; but a 'harsh and dreadful thing.'

Greater good, community good, individual good. Lesser evil.

Neat solution. Untidy non-solution. Resolving things. Living with things beyond resolving.

What to do?

. . .

Let us pursue this good man, the Father Abbot, as he pursues the always elusive thing to be done.

Several things. First, let us end this secrecy, which thrusts the consciences of us all in a closet; and turns the key.

Is the community composed of children, to be protected at all costs, and I the paterfamilias of their consciences? Rubbish! Have done with it.

Father Abbot?—or brother abbot?

I consider within myself the convenience and tidiness of the present arrangement; me as father, they as sons (adolescent, or preadolescent). How neat, how beneficial to both sides!

No more of it. This I will do. Tell them. Trust them.

Then let us make a proffer to our afflicted brother. Let him, by all means, remain. We urge it, we want him among us.

The law? Let him remain, if he so chooses, and within the law.

Which is to say, let him remain in the status he now holds. Neither novice nor monk; but postulant. One who is inside the door, one of us. As fully as can be, under the circumstances.

In this way, with the canny aiming of one stone, several birds will come to ground. I have overcome the plague of secrecy, by entrusting to the community a difficult news. I have even appealed to them; not to leave me alone with this anguish. Help me, so that we may help our brother.

I have also put the law in its rightful place. Which is to say, not the final arbiter of conscience, the word set in stone, and we indentured to it. No, but a light on our path; a path we must clear even as we walk.

And what if they refuse, what if such a solution is beyond them, and they decide . . . he must go?

We shall take that as it comes.

. . .

Thus my ruminations, a fiction, set down as though they were fact.

Alas, as events unrolled, sane alternatives were scuttled. Secrecy prevailed. The postulant was sent packing. The monks were informed only after the event, after the decision—in which they had been granted no part.

All this was accompanied, larded over with infinite civilized regret. The gate closed. But who issued free, and who were indentured in that closure, remains a cloud over those premises, a cloud in the unlikely form of a question mark.

. . .

It should be added; I do not mean, in the above reflections, to stigmatize the monks. There is little reason to believe that in similar circumstances, any order of men (including my own), confronted with a like dilemma, would not act in similar fashion. We all habitually cower under the law, our cover and heal-all, our very catoptric, the light we seek light by.

. . .

It stings, the memory of that rejection.

Aley died, I recounted the episode to friends. They were in varying degree appalled.

. . .

We sit at a coffee house table, my diminutive friend and I. His eyes are filled with pain. Mine—if eyes were hands, I would take his face in my hands, and make his pain my own.

There is a communion, as palpable as the breaking of bread. By an act of God we have passed from being children of this world, born of it, indebted to it—to another status. We are its bare survivors. We have graduated out of—better, been thrust out of—the world's 'elements,' as Paul describes them.

Thrust out of the law, in the first instance. Lawless.

Lawless, in favor of the great law, the first law. The law commended by Jesus. Love one another.

We had not known, as children of this world (children of the church of this world), the cost of this seemingly easeful command. It rolls so easily off the tongue, it trips from the mouth, it is one of the sonorous themes of mindless homilists.

Cleanse my lips, O Lord, who cleansed the lips of the prophet Isaiah with a burning coal; that I may proclaim your word.

. . .

I've met others before, on that plateau where for the time being, all seems well.

Aley is on AZT, the newest chemical wonder. Every four hours, night and day, he pops the pills.

As with every wonder and its works, there is a reckoning. In his case, though the 'Big D' has ceased wracking him, his appetite has also fled. So the weight loss must be countered. Also, his blood must be tested regularly, since the wonder drug, in process of working its wonders, tends also to diminish the white corpuscles.

For every gain, a loss. But the gain, for now, by far outweighs the loss. He's in good fettle, though fragile.

It's called life on the raft, in mid-sea. Seas, for the moment, tranquil. But (we needn't tell him, he knows it) the barometer is falling.

. . .

Nagasaki day, 1988. The city is blanketed in a damp, smoggy gloom, dawn to noon to dusk, no perceptible alteration of light. The sun makes a reluctant appearance, the lordly Hudson sends forth breezes. Then it is as though a furnace door had opened to a throaty yell; more fuel!

Do we dwell, lucky denizens, near an ocean, and athwart two rivers? Are we not lucky islanders, Venetians of a new world? To no avail. Torment; we might well be staked to four corners of the Arizona desert.

Life; 'a painted ship upon a painted ocean.'

It is the forty-third anniversary of the atomic slaughter of Nagasaki. Along with some twenty-five other intransigent souls, I am arrested at the Riverside Research Institute. We have been detained there previously—how many times? Our stubborn wills reach back and back, to a first 'No,' uttered by Dorothy Day, within a week after the bomb fell.

. . .

Once released from (temporary) durance vile, I phone Aley. His velvet tones waft back, weaker than accustomed.

'The doctors said it may be anemia, due to the AZT. This morning they called to say it was so. I must have a blood transfusion.'

The arrest in the summer heat, the ride across Manhattan in the police chariot, have left me limp indeed. We are, for the moment, in something like the same condition. I not apt for a visit, he lethargic. We agree to wait for the morrow.

The differences in our respective statuses escape neither of us. I am in no need of infusion of blood. Indeed on many occasions, I have disposed of superfluous rubrical riches, by pouring them out—whether at the pentagon or at the Riverside laboratories or elsewhere.

This has been a peculiar source of satisfaction. It is as though my friends and I have been blessed by an invitation; to transfuse our blood in the neediest of bodies; in that body of the military, where the subject of blood is seldom mentioned and invariably, immemorially in the air. Giving of blood? Hardly; much shedding of blood.

. . .

Any of us would beyond doubt shed our blood for Aley's benefit. Perhaps we are already doing so.

Recent converse with him, as the city swelters and sweats, is limited to the telephone.

Weak he may well be, but his talk pours out nonetheless. Good news and bad, the invariable mix.

Anemia indeed confirmed . . . brought on by the new drugs. Saturday he'll repair to the hospital for a transfusion.

He's jubilant for another reason. He has come on a better place to live. 'In the south of Manhattan; so I'll be close to the hospital and doctors.'

And how had the proffer come about? He was put on the trail by an ad in the *Village Voice*. Talked with the landlord, whose duplex he'll be welcomed into.

Then the crasher; 'He has AIDS too.'

Aley's decision to move made a kind of sense in the mad times. I hastened to bless his decision. 'This is wonderful news; you'll each be great help to the other.'

'His lover died in the spring. He's been looking for someone ever since. The place is comfortable, I'm going to take it.'

I can almost feel on the wire, the beat of his pulse grows stronger.

Then more good news. He's gotten wind of a holistic doctor in New York who treats AIDS patients. Will see him for the first time in two days. Who can tell, maybe he'll be able to toss all the 'wonder drugs' in the ash can.

. . .

Late September, the weather at last tempering. He came to dinner. The six guests were charmed out of their pelts by his incandescent talk. His eyes danced a fandango in his head, as he held forth on his latest trip, two weeks at his erstwhile monastery in Georgia.

The message from that mysterious lamasery seemed to be (as far as one can make sense of such goings on)—you're always welcome, as you understand. As a guest.

He arrived, as a guest. Was asked abruptly by the brother who conveyed him from the airport, 'Are you going to try to return?' Quite a welcome.

But was a genius at evoking our sorry best. Said, eyes alight, in those liquid Latin tones; 'It was just like a family, we had our differences, and had them out. I asked the Father Prior whether he thought it was the Christian thing to do, sending me home because I had AIDS. He got all flustered, and shouted at me; it's canon law, I'm helpless.

'The father also asked, was I receiving encouragement from the brothers to apply again? He said, if they're doing so, they're raising false hopes. These are exactly the ones who would vote against you if it came to that.

'He went on: It wouldn't be fair in any case, to yourself, if we were to admit you. You have to be so careful of your health, to impose our rule would be a cruelty.'

. . .

I said nothing.

But questioned my soul; aren't we supposedly liberated from the law, in virtue of the life and death of Christ? And does not a sane view of any rule regard it as a norm, a guide, a kind of light on the path—not the path itself, let alone the goal? The mind boggles.

Aley: 'You have so many admirers down there. They wonder why you don't come for a visit.'

I: 'It's because of you.'

Subject closed.

. . .

He looked wonderfully restored, ate with gusto. I was delighted.

After dinner, he produced a few photos. In the monastery he had been a designer and maker of stained glass. (Of this phase of his life, he had told me nothing.)

The work was exquisite. One window portrayed Jesus and Mary, hands intertwining, affection, respect, access, distance.

Aley has a canny way of astonishing one; up his sleeves are card tricks, doves, coins out of thin air, rabbits. He had talked of his novitiate tasks; they always seemed quite humdrum, the make-work they assign to novices, or the drudge's assignments that are rotated among everyone.

I surmise he'd taken his turn at that too, laundry, floor scrubbing. But this!

. . .

The long nights crept in. It was Christmas time. I held a party to celebrate ... what? The return, meager and scarcely to be sensed, of that light we call hope.

It will not do, I thought, in such a season, to sit about licking one's wounds—which by everyone's admission, have multiplied in the past year.

In the guests came, Aley in their midst. But with a notable change about him, and hardly for the better; feverish, untowardly quiet in manner. He was weak of frame and white of face, his color blanched, his eyes glittering.

Yet he had come to celebrate with us. Damn the fever, full speed ahead.

I learned in the course of the evening, he eating and drinking by sheer will—learned that the fever had been burning for some days.

But no complaints; only a factual stating of the case. And the voice purred on, caressing vowels, merest touch and go upon consonants. Concerning his friends, concerning visits and events, his socializing here and there in past weeks.

An inconsequential sweetness masking a great courage, a purpose undeclared; the drawing of death's sting.

You have to be Latino, I said to my inner soul, you have to touch as lightly upon life and death (your own life and death) as you do upon the peck of pickled peppers, the hisses, the p's and t's that spit, spiky from Anglo lips.

Lightly, lightly, easy rider. Love life so passionately you give it up—passionately.

I played sedulous host, a weather eye out, second servings and so on. All to the good, all normal.

And no swooning diva he, no special case.

Goodnight at the door. He embraced me as though some message were pressing home. I said without knowing why: 'I want to hear from you every day for awhile; how things are going, whether the fever is under control.'

And he, half humorous, wholly serious; 'You'll hear from me all right.' And then a toss over his shoulder, with a grin; 'You'll never be rid of me.'

. . .

Now and again my prophetic bones groan in their sockets. A day or so later word came; 'He's in hospital, we're very worried, he's not responding to treatment.'

Which he wasn't, as was plain, even shocking to the eye. No spate of greeting, his spirit was listless, guttering in the wind.

He was in shock, I thought. He didn't expect this blow, so hard, so quick. He knew a decline would at some point set in. But he'd be in command, dignity intact, going out on his own terms.

Alas and alack, it never happens that way.

. . .

They go like this, the last days;
—The illness breaks the heart, you all but hear the breaking of bones.
—At some point, self-command turns to a great fiction.
—Now you're at the mercy of your bowels rampant, your pisser geysering like Old Faithful, your failing eyes or limbs or ... mind.
—Toward the end you crawl about like a Kafkaesque bug.
—Then you've only the absurd rectangle of a bed to toss about in.
—You no longer retain food, you spit and vomit bile.
—Comes a time when you crap your sheets to a fare-thee-well, you turn in your own sodden filth, until someone (not prompt, not cheerful, only hired to do the work no one else will put hand to) appears; or does not appear.
—The knees cave in, the machinery is stalled.

And you're still, as they say, living.

. . .

He looked well attended to, peaceable, wistful, the ghost of former days. It's called, in terms borrowed for the skin trade, slippage. He was coming unmoored, a tide was sucking him toward the open sea.

He was at the mercy of a love whose direction is . . . Unknown.

Visitors came and went, I came and went. It was hard, hard; we were so used to bibbing at this bright fountainhead of good spirits—waiting for his lead, his gentle witticisms and unexpected turns and detours—we had only to play the minor part, captivated.

. . .

Were we not the audience of a full-scale drama, three acts or five and a classical, logical outcome, neat as the dovetailing of a wing?

How ill prepared we were for the end, the botch on stage, the curtain rattling down. The house manager, embarrassed, appears at the footlights, his words faltering on his stuck tongue; Ladies, gentlemen, to the infinite regret of the house. . . .

It was drama as deception, the overthrow of that cozy providence we had leaned on like infants: to, fro, in the Everlasting Arms.

That face, that figure distorted and flickering in the wings. It was Pirandello, turning the game to a farce, turning the gods' pockets inside out.

We raged—and we knew. It was curtains; we shuffled heavy-footed and leaden of heart toward the exit.

Opening night, and the play closed like a locked jaw. How could it go on, the star lying dead in mid-act?

FIVE

PETER AND CARY AND THE THIRD PARTY LURKING

I carry about with me an abiding dread; that the dying of friends be made 'presentable.'

This, I hasten to add, is far from a majority sentiment. According to the standards of American Hecatomb Corp., which arranges for the denigrating departure of most of us, only death itself is presentable.

'We don't care what went before' is roughly the motto. How badly you look as you lie there, how mottled, how desiccated, how unpresentable—'Fear not! The hateful passage made, we shall make you—the absent you, the sweet dry shell of you, the approximate you—pumped up, paradisiacal, presentable!'

The promise is Dantesque-grotesque. The scene, one thinks, could only be Infernal.

Now in one sense (the only one that makes sense to me) exactly the opposite is the truth. Death, de facto death, death as relic, sere leaf, a corpse, its time served—none of this is of any abiding interest.

. . .

It is the dying of my friends that is eminently presentable. Presentable, and then some; before God and those who attend them. The dying of friends being a presentment and reminder of the stories, hints, traditions, images of the dying of the saints. And of that One whose dying the Saints point to, like a field of wheat bent by an overriding wind, a sudden epiphany.

And that dying, despite most contemporary (and inevitably technological) evidence to the contrary, remains a hard chore indeed.

Let it be said clearly (the saying issues from the undergoing). Dying isn't a light show in a tunnel, Grandma's face by Whistler, a forest of arms incanting happy homecoming, turkey on the table, California massage or Southern Comfort. None of these.

On this subject, which is comparable to a moral twilight zone, any sharp semblance of night, real night, or day, real day, would come as a species of relief. The Savior's agon might thus offer some light; or some darkness.

His dying, as the four evangelists are agreed, could only be described as horror, disgrace, loss, anguish, desolation, abandonment. There is no point enlarging on the original accounts, which speak of a sublime spirit, discharged from this world in an explosion of pain, obloquy, and official contempt.

We have little evidence to shore up the cultural assurances, which have about them the spurious sleazy comfort of a Dickensian mortician.

A nightmare might help our understanding; or a daymare. Dying is a little like finding oneself straddling the continental shelf, one foot east, one foot west. Suddenly the plates start to groan and grieve underfoot. Your body, trying for all hell to hold on, east and west, splits like a wishbone.

Now what part of me wins, what loses? Can part of anyone win and another part lose? And when the cosmic perturbation subsides, where do we (or is it I?) stand? Is east still east, west west?

. . .

I should know, I've been there. I was in prison in 1970-72, for daring to suggest that the war in Vietnam was not our finest hour. And for daring to dramatize, along with eight other intemperate souls, our heart's conviction. The crime is admitted, your honor. Stipulated. Here's how it went, your honor. We took out some draft files from an obscure rickety draft center in Maryland (draft files, like the poor enrolled there, are seldom luxuriously housed) and burned the 'hunting licenses against humans' with napalm we had concocted in someone's kitchen.

Indeed we did, your honor. And that, to put the matter felonious and short, was our finest hour. No qualifying, no kidding.

So all nine of us landed in prison, except David Darst. He by a particularly lousy twist of fate (that lousy clone of faith) landed in . . . eternity. Killed in a motor accident and consequent freeway fire.

RIP, dear brother, these many years.

I, meantime, and the other seven, survived.

This survival story (bare survival really) is about me. The only reason for telling it is the subject, survival.

. . .

I escaped death by a hair's breadth. It was a dental accident. I had been assigned to the dental clinic by a system which, I was told in all sorts of ways, was anxious to rehabilitate me.

The axiom was historically prior to the later statement of intent by the same system; to wit, the purpose of the justice system (or the prison system, twins of one egg) was to punish me.

No matter, they rehabilitated like hell, they punished like hell. In the system, rehab was one with punish; and vice versa. You were not required to know this; you were better off if you didn't.

Indeed, watch out; the knowledge might well inhibit the effect.

I got something of the latter, and only enough of the former, as not to adhere for long. This is a true confession.

Meantime they almost killed me. This event was a bit more disturbing than punishment or rehabilitation. It was, moreover, not included in the scenario of crime and punishment. Who, I asked myself at the time, as I dazed about in the twilight zone—who were they to decree when and/or where I was to meet my Maker?

The dentist had pumped me full of some patented pain killer, trying to render his next move, a particularly awful filling, bearable.

It is perhaps worth noting that I was not only his patient, I was (though beyond the pale, a prisoner), I was his colleague, so to speak.

And within minutes following his injection, I was dying. It was simple and clean as that. Everything—heart, lungs—slowed, then halted. The dentist summoned others of his kind, they got me horizontal, brought my brother Phil racing in from the far side of the compound.

It was, I judge, another one of those finest hours. I was walking out of an unenviable terrain, free. Crime? Punishment? Death came like the angel in Acts that nudged Peter, a prisoner. Get up, he said. And doors opened. Because, it was said, the church was at prayer for him.

You never know, angels take the weirdest forms. Sometimes, they say, angels of death.

. . .

As to this friend of mine. The common assumption is taken quite matter-of-factly on his part. The assumption; only a little time is left to him. Also the grief; quite matter-of-factly (to all appearances). He's already lost his lover of many years.

A phrase comes to mind; nobility of grief. And more grief impending. And in view of that weight, lowering itself ponderously to his shoulders, he summons a greater nobility.

I am instructed, reminded, dazzled.

In our novitiate days, we were exposed to a tome of spiritual discipline whose structure went this way; first, 'The Teaching,' then 'The Foregoing Illumined by Examples.'

. . .

As in the instance of Peter.

I meet him on a wintry day in an overheated apartment in Chelsea, Manhattan. His demesne is a walkup of four flights. A century ago, the building was a slum or immigrant dwelling; recently, in a manner of speaking common to landlord jargon, it has been renovated, upgraded. The subject is $$$.

Upgrade? Even according to New York standards of unblemished greed (bleed the tenant, do the least, get the most)— the so-called improvement is beyond doubt minimal. The rugs that crawl the stairway are soiled and smelly; the stairs themselves narrow as a landlord's eye, tipsy as the deck of a catastrophe-prone ocean liner.

You climb and climb, listing a little as you go. At length, courage shaken, you enter the apartment of a working man. He's been, in palmier days, a carpenter and builder. Craggy face, big prow of a nose, chin firm, mouth generous. The physique of one who has put muscle to bending, sawing, planing, the right use of tools, transforming metals and woods into usefulness and beauty.

And how he loves to talk! Not any talk at all, not the kind that comes and goes, from nowhere to elsewhere. He loves good talk; seeks it out, evokes it, creates it. Spontaneity and verve, headlong.

And a gift for friendship. As I was to learn, to my sorrow and joy, in the months that followed. He knew something of the list of the world, and the crazy stairway that led, only now and then, to a realm of sanity. He knew how seldom friends announced themselves in his place, in the time A. D. (After the Dires), how friendship paled and quite vanished under the news no one wanted to hear; but he must.

A Southerner from a poor family. Much praise of his grandmother, who raised him, his mother having in his infancy 'given me away.' I hadn't heard that phrase before.

I was to meet this woman one day face to face, and see in her eyes something seldom seen on the planet; eyes turned to ice in a face turned to adamant.

. . .

On the walls were a series of sketches of women's fashions, the work of his new roommate.

Peter strikes me as—sound. He's firmly planted in his convictions; it's as though his heart had free voice.

'What I remember about Grandma, she had value, and stuck by it. She honored good work, and being really alive; a sense of others, come good or bad. She did her own housework and cooking well after eighty. And she tol' me again and again, If you're going to do something worthwhile with your life, then do it, and keep doin' it! Til it's done! That's the way the Lord calls us, work fit to be called His work.'

* * *

You wouldn't think, from the look of him, that he's so ill. As far as appearances go, nothing has sapped or zapped him. (As yet; it's always as yet in this game.) A worker's compact physique, big in shoulders and chest, small in waist. No sign as yet of the horror that lurks.

Ah, appearances! His hair sits close on his skull; chemotherapy struck at the roots, but his crowning glory is creeping back, fine as black moss.

And now he's ingesting the mysterious AZT.

He's had no carpentry jobs for some nine months. Been 'lazing it,' he says wryly. He's been in hospital or back in this darkened little room, music or TV blaring away. 'Sometimes you couldn't believe it, I'm just too weak to look at the damn tube. My head rolls to one side, and fore I know it, I'm out.'

It's all said without a trace of complaint; as though he's reporting on someone else.

* * *

He wonders aloud, what lies beyond death, by implication his own. 'I don't have any sense at all that those who died are able to give me some kind of hint as to my future, wherever. What do you think?'

I tell an episode out of our family. How according to strong belief, our mother, long dead, continues her care of us. How her prayers, as we believe, have brought about an altogether unexpected reconciling among the sons. An achievement that, left to ourselves and our sorry devices, we couldn't have brought to pass in an aeon; and yet it happened.

More; I think Peter's own supple and effervescent spirit is a hint; something of a power beyond the ordinary. I say so. He listens intently, but I sense that to his way of thinking, I tend to the needless complication of simple matters.

What could be simpler, or more to be taken for granted, than that one would face death courageously (he spreads his hands, the gesture says it all)—rather than glowering or complaining or making things impossible for those around?

He has a point; but the point flows from his own innocence and strength.

And all the while, of his own gifts he's blessedly unaware.

Somewhere about lurks the ghost of that wondrous grandma, her down home dicta in his ear.

'Be what you're going to be, she tol' me, the best around. And no one has to know it, it's just there. Funny thing, if you're right and straight and have no bones to pick, it won't be long afore they know it; and then some. Then comes the respect, and that's worth it all.'

. . .

He had voyaged to Central America and taught school there, has wandered up and down the southern cone. Can discourse at length, and does, on the cultures and customs of people he moved among.

Was an alcoholic and drug addict for years, lived a derelict life on the streets, came back from it.

Then this.

. . .

You don't hear a sound, the skies fall in ever so sweetly and finally. It's like the last day of a cosmos.

Or like the collapse of the Great Wall of China. It starts so simply, hardly noticed. One night a few bricks, loosened by age and frost, fall. Fifty years later, something more; a section weakens, leans over. Then ever so slowly a long ribbon, miles long, up hill and down dale, curls and turns about, a dragon stricken.

And all in an immense slowness, a kind of regal dignity—like an emperor silently buckling and falling in his coronation robes.

· · ·

'It comes to this; you're next to dead, and it's happening so slow or so fast you can't tell which. It's over 'fore you know it's got to you. You're falling, falling, it's the longest nightmare since Adam lost Eden. You're vertical, dead, an' you haven't hit ground.'

Friends are long gone, the family for the most part ashamed and silent. They hide out. What's happened, AIDS? Sorry, we don't know the gent.

Then the shock passes, to a degree. The fallen dominoes pick themselves up; some of them. But when they've reassembled, it's a new game. Former friends, former family. Former church. So many people backing away! They've bought oxen or leased farms or married, as the gospel has it. The message to the sufferer is clear; get lost.

Among some of those 'formers,' an added insult is proffered; P.S. We'll pray for you.

· · ·

I submit this; anybody who copes with the above, forbids himself bitterness or rancor, even while he feels his gorge rising and hands twitching for a throat—such a one deserves the crown of a saint, on the spot.

(Which, it goes without saying, isn't likely, in casu. The Saint makers being, so to speak, occupied with dishing out those polluted prayers for the eternal benefit of such sinners as you know who.)

. . .

Peter isn't greatly afflicted with such morbidities of spirit.

'There's kinds of religion tailor-made to drive you insane. Among which, Southern Baptist takes the front rank. I saw it, I walked away, early on. Wanted to stay sane; or failing that, go insane my own way.'

We sit there in the frumpy front room, the unmade bed against the window, the stereo thumping and wailing. He serves a cup of tea. The dog waddles in and commences a big affectionate drooly fuss. Peter points out, with the faintest touch of longing and loss, this or that piece of furniture, the work of his hands; a weighty marble shelf above the fireplace, a table on casters that doubles as storage space. No mean artisan he.

Tools laid down, for good. 'The things I did in my prime! Haven't been able to build anything for months, here or anywhere else.'

. . .

Now and then, things get plain hilarious.

Peter and a friend, Cary, were to come to 98th Street for dinner one night; cooked by me. This might seem hardly worth recording, except for this: in Peter's mind, it was an enterprise of stupendous proportions. Thirty blocks by cab, from his door to mine.

Since his illness, he'd become a hearth cat, a faunum curled about the amenities of TV and rock music, loud enough to split an oak log.

Thus we reconnoitered and juggled matters, by phone. First it was yes they would come for supper, then no they wouldn't. Finally (or so it seemed), to fro and to once more, they would.

It was the coldest night of the year; I had qualms and rode the acceptance lightly, knowing Peter was housebound by more than simple choice. He was habitually congested, weakened by his long-drawn-out illness.

The witching hour approached, the groaning board groaned.

And he was on the horn once more. His friend had not yet arrived from work, though he had promised to appear a half-hour before. Therefore and ergo they would not, could not come to dinner.

Further ramifications, another call. Now it was the friend, professing his misunderstanding of the hour of dinner, etc., etc. He was chastened, he regretted, etc.

The upshot, they did not come. The board groaned deeper, as though from the guts of The Fat Man, with plenty, with loss. Thanksgiving Day approaches, I said to my soul, We'll try again.

. . .

The smallest ray of insight would disclose the story and its nobility. By no means a frivolous vocation; to live with a very ill friend, day after day to bear with the inevitable, to keep one's courage and spirit intact, coping meantime with job, with cooking, shopping, cleaning; with one's own swing of mood.

With New York. Cary, friend of Peter, someone worth knowing!

. . .

The two did of course eventually come to dinner, and more than once. The events were so arranged that several of my community met them around the table.

And on at least one occasion, an exchange took place, the like of which my Jesuit guests seldom or never are exposed to.

What did it mean to face one's own death, within a year of the death of one's lover? How, in Peter's own estimation, was he coping with such dire events?

Deep waters, chill, and . . .

Then Cary; he had entered Peter's life, he became the wage earner of the duet. 'And the cook as well,' he interjected, half humorously, half in indignation. 'And the shopper, and just for the record, the dish washer too!'

For Peter, life was summed up in a flat facing of 'things as they are.' And more; 'getting to one's resources, I mean spiritually. You have to have something goin' for you. Otherwise the bottom drops out of life; "why go on" becomes yer whine.'

Cary, such burdens taken on, has grown. 'I think to myself, what is one to do with his life, except give and give? And stick with someone, thick and thin? I'm a tribal person, my background is Polynesian. We're big on family. In lonely New York, I have to have someone to come home to. This is grief, but also privilege.'

And so on, each in that vein.

The Jesuits were bug-eyed.

I think we saw our own community in a light that shamed us, and at the same time, opened a vein of hope.

. . .

I urged on the two a vacation from the city; offered them a week at Block Island in the cottage. There was much verbal to and fro on this. Peter is morbidly attached to his couch, his turf, his four walls. How bestir him?

All sorts of objections; the long train trip, the transfer to auto and plane.

A friend made an offer to chauffeur them in his car; then the offer fell through.

Result; no result. They will stay put, come what torrid days there may. And will. Such days (daze) as indeed are presently being laid upon us, as the city stokes up, a vast steaming cauldron.

. . .

I made my way frequently that summer to the doggy apartment. There emanated from floors and walls the effects of a canine, generally hirsute decor. It was compounded, as in certain esoteric 'total sensory films,' by an ambiguous appeal to smell, sight, touch, clamorous hearing—and by way of vapors and inhalation, even taste. No part or power spared.

Thus we sat, amid the most persuasive evidence that we were, if anything, the secondary inhabitants of the place. The dog, as 'environmental impact' indicated, was the primary situant; we the guests.

It was like a medieval mystery play, meant to instruct and entertain both, a minuscule illustration of cosmic event.

. . .

A stately herald opens the drama. Consider our estate, he intones, splendid in his lozenged attire, half jester, half wizard. For we are also guests upon the earth, briefly tottering and reeling about, for the most part off balance.

More; indentured and debtors. It is forbidden to think of ourselves as permanent owners, denizens, disposers, of ... anything; apartments, accouterments. No, we are tolerated and grinned at; even by canines.

I enter into these daunting matters, mostly by way of setting a contrasting tone. Our conversation, Peter's and mine, is invariably quite matter-of-fact. We talk as though we were composing out of thin air and wit a good short story; withholding its clue, readying the whiplash at the end.

. . .

We got into a routine of sorts. He invariably made coffee, I brought along a box of favorite cookies available in the neighborhood. We sat there in the heat, hardly relieved by an asthmatic air conditioner.

That room! Cluttered and dowdy, redeemed by the presence of a friend, a conscientious refuser of the Great Induction.

The heat fell on us like the blows of a triphammer, day after day. Our talk grew desultory, matters of little or no moment. We were like those who wait and wait; some matter of great moment, a curtain call perhaps, a first night.

Meantime ... a meantime.

And someone keeping time; a Third Party Lurking.

. . .

I was out of town for some weeks, teaching in New Orleans; then we connected again.

My friend was much altered in appearance and diminished in spirit. He leaned back, brushed aside my inquiries, peremptorily (and beyond his custom) with a dismissive shake of the head. Enough of state of health; he turned to other matters.

I was puzzled. In the past he had been candid, even voluble, about his condition, his chances.

. . .

Today he would rather dwell on small matters than large. Our talk meandered along; the heat of the day, from which he was sensibly delivered by keeping to his room; the heat of the jungle I had endured in making the film "The Mission," an ordeal brought to mind only too vividly in mad New York July. Thence to his memories of Guatemala and El Salvador, his teaching stint. The wonderful artifacts of those countries, the present plight of their Indian peoples.

So it went.

I said my adieu, and made for the door. We would meet again shortly, words were exchanged about a dinner at my place.

Then, as I stood and bade goodbye, came the bolt of lightening, sheer white, it lit his face in the gloom. 'Sit down, please. I want to talk about my funeral.'

. . .

I sat again, slowly.

'What do you have to offer a non-Catholic like me? You know my lover was Catholic; I'd like to have something like what yew call a Mass. Can we?'

On my assurance that yes, we could; 'Then where is it to be, we have to think of these things. I'll talk it over with Cary. And yew know' (this with all seriousness and pathos) 'he's going to need some friendship an' help after I'm gone.'

There it was again, the heart of the matter; that thought of the other. Cary has to be prepared. Cary has to be helped face things. 'Ah've always understood these religious doins are more for the sake of the livin' than of departed. No?' Thank you good man, indeed so.

· · ·

There were days when I lost track of him, as of a planet in a changeful sky. Phone calls in vain. An answering machine giving back a raucous burst of rock music, then a ghostly simulacrum of his voice.

I kept trying; there was little else to do.

Finally an answer, feeble. 'Hullo.' A mere echo of an echo.

That old nemesis of the ill had seized on him and away he went, to hospital. Liquid had collected in his guts; he must be tapped like a wine barrel.

'Wal, they went at it, tried this an' that. Oh, those needles. Of course they're afraid of internal bleeding.'

It was a waiting game. 'Came the weekend, the hospital rolls over an' goes dead. It meant hangin' around in that room through Monday, then they start hemming an' hawing all over again, what to try next.

'Trouble is they're trained to deal with conventional stuff, don't know beans about death-dealing illness. Them doctors! If you had someone dying on your hands, would you leave town for the weekend?'

He'd taken things in his own hands. 'More I thought about it, less sense it made. So come Friday evening I up an' signed myself out. Out an' home sweet home.'

It wasn't elegant, it wasn't according to Hoyle or the rules of the medical game. It was only ... crucial. He'd reclaimed his soul. He'd so often said it; what time was left belonged to him—not to doctors or their 'procedures.'

. . .

He often spoke of dignity. The usage was not only the message; one couldn't miss the mode, the slow speech, the direct look out as he fingered his cigarette and the smoke went up unwavering. You met his eye, his met yours through the haze. Slow motion; slow in everything except moral understanding. That was fast and firm indeed.

I talk with him about young Cary; I talk with the nursing team. We're all puzzled and a bit apprehensive. What's going on with that feisty spirit, what will go on as things worsen and Peter lies there, tossed hither and yon by the rip tide? We don't know, we can't do much except stand by.

. . .

Come on up for supper, both of you.
But it's no go, not up to it, too weak, etc.
Well, then, I'll tool down to your lair during the week.
He seems at peace with that.

. . .

I venture again through the corridors and up the stairs. A veritable rite of passage, the immigrant's 'walk-up.' The hallway an unsteady riot of tile, as though a design of sorts were flung down randomly from on high. Discolored rug crawling the stair, local grit, sweat, mud, an all-weather index of the passage of mortal beings. A ladder of sorts, no heaven in sight.

It is as though Grandfather Time mounted the steps, armed with his summons, knocking on doors.

On each landing, a cultural relic of note. First, a large plantain in a pot, some four feet in height; and appended, a torn scribbled notice; DO NOT REMOVE. The neck of the plant is sagging. I am not convinced that the bedraggled, indeed terminal condition of the florum would of itself arouse cupidity. Especially as the heft of it might be thought excessive by all except a crew of dockmen.

I continue up. On the next landing, a gas stove squats. A sign warning off interlopers; DO NOT ET CETERA. I am warned off.

Next landing, Peter's, and a more welcome emblem. Between the narrow walls two large framed maps are hung. Each faces the other, complementary versions of the universe. The colors are reassuring as mutual smiles. A map of New York harbor, another, the world of some unknown cartographer of the seventeenth century. Find your way, through time, through this world.

. . .

Cary greets me at the door. This is the first surprise. He has never been found lingering on the premises during a 'work day.'

'How come?'

'Oh, well, the weather is so awful, who wants to work today?'

I have a suspicion. Both have endured the recent awful hospital episode, together with its ominous undetermined outcome. They want me there, to talk things out. Cary makes coffee, we settle in.

The heat is damnable.

Peter, alas, is sadly altered in appearance; belly distended, skin alarmingly pallid. He reviews his recent maltreatment at the hospital. I agree, the story is peculiar to New York, The City Where Things Are Awful, Invariably Tending To Awfuller.

The life (and death) of Peter will remain bearable, only if Cary is taken into account.

These are subtle matters, let alone painful. 'Who's dying?'

The answer, straight as a blast from the blunderbuss named time, is . . . Peter.

But who's got to survive, whose vocation is it to survive?

And who of us isn't aware that under some circumstances, survival can be a more terrible prospect than death?

In that room, that day, one heard only questions.

. . .

Cary aware . . . and unaware. Those wrinkles on nose and handsome forehead, the faraway look that takes over, as though he's looking beyond a present too painful to dwell on.

Aware and unaware. To the point, beside the point; we turn and twist on that terrible Archimedean point called death.

. . .

This and that on our tongues, the untidy little room, the smells and sounds, traffic outside, the fan, a bare pant of relief. We have coffee before us, time weaves its web, point to point, life to life, we three. We're surely, squarely planted in this world.

But no one of us is deceived; the world heaves underfoot, the world is composed of turbulent lava. We're survivors on an uneasy island, roughly the dimension of that four-square room.

. . .

More than one motive rides the stale air. Cary took a holiday because Peter is so ill, and because I'm coming by. Because all three of us are between hell and a hard place.

Because my brother Phil is in prison, and my brother Tom has suffered a stroke and heart attacks. Because months ago brother John was struck by a car and all but hamburgered. Because because.

Because we're clinging to one another for dear life, in this room. On mortality's rickety islet. Survivors.

Peter perks up.

We talk in fact, of practically anything . . . but death.

By design? Partly, I surmise. He and Cary want more time before unveiling the subject. An intricate choreography eventually will come together—but only toward the close.

. . .

Now this is passing strange. A kind of welcome is offered the kiss of death—so I can go on living. The kiss of death is bestowed on me by someone near death; a mouth or cheek or hand, whatever is offered.

So I might say to death, Kiss Off.

. . .

Another day. We talked awhile, then let the long silences take over. It was, so to speak, a seminar on Ways & Means of Hoping and Coping.

This wasn't in the nature of a new assignment. I'd been at it a long, long time, longer by far than those sitting with me, the young Polynesian innocent and the wise ex-alcoholic carpenter; 'they went to sea in a sieve. . . . '

One of them knew something, one knew much more. One was shortly to know it all.

Indeed quite a trinity.

. . .

Rarely, Peter would consent to depart his room in quest of whatever r. and r. might be available in the neighborhood. Such diversions were, by any standards, modest.

One time, he shepherded me into a chrome and linoleum emporium, a kind of truck stop apotheosized in favor of the new yuppie hierophants.

I ordered coffee, he an omelette, coffee and dessert. The bill was in the neighborhood of $18.00. I paid up, muttering through clenched teeth, never again.

. . .

He had a gustatory itch; chocolate cookies. I would stop at the neighborhood Party Cake. This center of delights lay in a forsaken wedge of Chelsea; around it, filthy Chinese booths dispensed cheap soup by the plastic cup. The street corners were crowded with the various colors and permutations of the Fruit of the Human Loom.

Party Cake Local tended toward the cozily inefficient and barely presentable. Elders of the neighborhood hung out over the sticky table tops, there was loud palaver concerning undecipherable, strictly insular doings; and delicious digs, followed by bellows of laughter. Everyone appeared to be in on the proffered joke, no matter its impermeability to the outsider.

I would line up at the counter to procure Peter's treat.

His taste tended toward the catholic; generous, but within limits; to wit, anything chocolate.

Eventually, a languishing attention would be paid my presence. One of several nearly inert girls would drift in my direction, the chief point of interest being not the customer, but the telephone, which must reluctantly be abandoned in favor of the interloping seeker of sweets. Outgoing calls, be it added.

. . .

I was away briefly. And as usual, haunted by apprehension. How was he faring?

I need not have worried. When I returned he was in an uncanny holding pattern. Holding his weight, his appetite— his own, as they say.

The usual amenities were served. We briefly discussed his health; the indirections were remarkably direct. He came to the point; his hopes for 'my last days.'

'Above all, I don't wanna be kept on machines, maybe I've said this before. No hooking me up. Please.'

'Here's how I see it. Let them drug me to the eyeballs, keep me in lala land, maybe a sniff of oxygen, nothing more. Then one day a week, bring me down. A few hours seeing my friends, saying goodbye, things like that, then let 'em waft me off again. And so go. And good luck everybody.'

. . .

In the event, the instruction did not hold. Not in the least. We were to see, weeks down the road, how he changed, how he signed papers and in consequence machines were hooked up, how he struggled like a tiger in a net.

But for a time, it seemed he'd leapt the barrier.

. . .

I tell him of my recent visit to London, the workshops in nonviolence.

Also of my visit to her majesty's prison known wondrously as 'Wormwood Scrubs,' and the prisoners known as the Birmingham Six. How I found two of them in fine fettle, though fourteen years have passed since their trial and conviction.

He listens in silent complicity. He knew it, one doesn't cross oceans to flee human misery or to punch up one's academic standing.

The cigarette smoke sits heavy on the sultry air. The weather is desperately humid; the sun day after day stokes the city. The air conditioner fritters and frets and relieves matters hardly at all. 'My electric bill last month was $240.00,' he observes laconically. 'That thing in the window must be leaking Con Ed's life blood.'

'Yours, more likely.'

'You said it. Then some.'

I speak of Berrigan family woes. Philip in jail. Tom ill with stroke and heart condition. John struck down in the street.

And now Jerry, and a cornea transplant. What a circle of Jobs we've become of late!

His sympathy is manifest. Not a word of his own supremely greater trouble. And I'm chastened.

. . .

Another day and up the staircase, the usual smells; doggy, catty, fishy, pissy. The shambles of a hallway. Peter at the door.

He looks . . . terrible, like a human cave-in; so much ground lost in so short a time. My heart does a pratfall.

He puts on a brave face.

There is the usual report (everything is usual, which is to say, catastrophic). Am I still in need of instruction—that urban events, at least according to the hornbooks thrust into my hands, lean toward—catastrophe? O slow learner!

He staggers to his feet in quest of coffee.

We sit and sip. The talk ranges from Central America to the idolatries of the presidential charade, all Bush league and Greek comico-tragico. He avers at one point that Bush ought in a sane society to be indicted for deceit: 'As if that could ever be considered a crime in this land. But he's committing a crime every day he opens his mouth.'

The talk turned desultory. And then, as sometimes happens with him, a chance observation brought me up short. He was discussing the nursing team from St. Vincent's.

'I don't know how they do it, day after day. At it since the early Eighties, dealing with all those deaths. And then the loss of John. . . . ' His voice trailed off.

My ears went erect. 'John who?'

'Why, I didn't tell you? The fellow we went out with two months ago to eat soul food.'

'He died?'

'Suicide. He no sooner got into his new place, so many people worked hard to find it. Then he did himself in.'

I remembered. Good God.

'Well, it was bound to come. A little gay kid who never grew up. He hung around here, I was tryin' for weeks to get him interested in doing something for others. Asked him how about going down to the gay men's health crisis folk an' help serve food to the ill? But no go.'

After an hour or more of this, he looks me straight in the eye, and starts.

'I want to talk about a funeral.'

He lit a cigarette. I required one.

'I've heard you talk with such love of that place, I want you to take my ashes to Block Island, an' scatter them in the sea, near the cottage.

'I want you to have a service too, with a few of my friends.

'You said it could be held at your apartment. That still stand?'

OK.

'I have Pierre's ashes in a box there in the corner. Please take his along an' pour us in the sea together. You pick the spot.' Then the grin. 'I want to swim in the ocean, off that island I never got to visit.'

It was time for a bit of lightness. 'I expect some return. You take over as guardian angel of the little house out there.'

'Agreed. And you'll take care of Cary afterward. He's really got no one else, losin' me will be losin' pretty near all he has.'

The nurse Kathy arrived. He went on tranquilly, continuing his instructions, as though in his eyes she were part of the picture; as indeed she is.

The talk turned to food. Kathy asked if I cooked. Pat interjected, 'He's a brilliant cook.'

'What's your speed?' she asked.

'Italian, thanks to my in-laws. And French, after living several years in Paris and elsewhere.'

'What do you cook for Peter and Cary?'

'First off I give thought to the guests. Meditate. Ask what they might likely enjoy. Usually I hit it right.'

Peter: 'He sure does.'

He broke off, as he often does, 'And of course I expect that my friends of the nursing team will come to my funeral.'

And the nurse: 'You can count on it.'

I stood to go. 'How about coming to my place for dinner on Sunday?'

'No appetite. We'll hafta see how I come out of this awful week.'

I cut out through the kitchen. Cary had arrived from work and was quietly cleaning up.

I repeated the invitation to dinner. He was sober, almost in tears. 'You're the only one who brings any help. He's down, more and more. Losing ground. Says he's tired of all this. And I don't blame him.'

Blame? I honor him with all my heart.

. . .

He used to look, I thought, sturdy as a king's guardsman, natty, neatly turned out by nature. He could cast a look that said: I own the future; and come to think of it, the present as well.

And now he's a near corpse. One doesn't need X-ray eyes to see him . . . dead.

One day, on the phone: 'Come on down, have a meal with us. Cary will get something together.'

Which, Sunday following, the good Cary did, bearing home a meal from the local Cubano 'home cooking' place.

The menu was somewhat short of spectacular; plastic and cardboard, the usual complement of takeout joints.

Nonetheless I sat down content to the improvised banquet of my beleaguered friends. Edgy as I was toward any claim on happiness (as they were too) knowing how near we trod to the edge of life. How short the time.

Having before us, in the one we loved, the evidence thereof.

Peter tried valiantly. He sat up and tried a few mouthfuls. No go. The pain sent him fainting backward against a pillow, face averted.

Meantime we made do, eating and drinking and nursing a meager converse. One eye on the viands, a wary weather eye on the suffering brother.

After a time he sat up, and said faintly; 'The pain's too much. Here goes with the drug.'

He imbibed a pill and sank back, with that look, wide-eyed and askance, that says, 'I'm a third party for the time being, leaving the first and second parties strictly to themselves. Meantime investigating another planet than yours, with a view toward entering an application for residence.'

Relief was late arriving. He moved to the bed, tried left side, then right, then positioned himself on his back; and finally, fretfully, groped for a cigarette; the gyrations of one in high fever or pain beyond bearing.

Suddenly the pain dissolved, the drug took him away. Then just as quickly he came back to us, glassily alert.

It was one of those chemical marvels, a kind of mirage. Anyone with good sense learns to distrust it, even as he marvels. I knew how dangerous it was, how passing and deceptive, with its white-hot flare of talk, its feverish insight, humor, the brain swinging about like a wrecking ball.

So we came to depend on pill popping for our converse. A new and ominous stage.

· · ·

As was to be proven.

. . .

Time grew short, the foreshortening seemed a very law of time, each segment shorter than the preceding. So that (in time), we would beyond doubt reach the geometric end of time.

Time was like a train, picking up passengers, baggage, as it lumbers and huffs along, station to station. Always shorter burdens at smaller stations. And finally in the darkness, we reach a desolate deserted platform, a single passenger, a nondescript morsel of baggage. And then sometime before dawn, welcome to a station that seems perpetually asleep.

No one mounts, no one descends. No coupling is in progress. Those who came aboard long before, sleep in darkened cars, behind lowered shades.

. . .

We sat in the raunchy untidy room, improvising out of cartons and plastic a meal. Outside the room—it seemed there was no outside, no noise, no strife. Only the smoke-stained windows, and across the way the tall canisters of misery, the public housing towers.

When I came out on the street an hour later, a full moon rode high, letting fall an aspergres of glory.

But in the apartment where Peter lay dying, no such solace touched us, no cataract of light blessed. We sat there, silent for the most part, in the foreshortened cube where death and dying cut corners sharp. We were learners in that austere box of a schoolroom; the lesson was four-square, take it or leave, and the ferule always at the ready. And on the dunce stools, one might imagine, sat the failed clowns who had badly construed the first lesson of all.

We were not failures. But neither were we graduates of that room, and its hard lessons.

He tossed about on his cot.

Finally he stirred, sat up and lit a cigarette.

Then like a latter day lazar, he rose unsteadily from the bed and made for the shelves where his books and photo albums lay in no discernable order.

'Who'd have thought,' he murmured, peering among the offerings, 'there'd come a day I could hardly make it across the room on my own two legs.'

Walk he did, as unlikely as Dr. Johnson's four-legged dog on two. He pulled down an album. 'Just take a look at this. I want you to see that little old shack I grew up in.'

There he was, a child no bigger than the weeds flourishing around him, sturdy in his pinafore, as though the weather of life were holding steady and bound to stay so.

Turning the pages, turning the years. He grinned through childhood like a halloween candle lit by an unknown hand. Then the smile turned to a knowing adolescent smirk; slick hair and tie and borrowed roadster and senior prom, the improvisations, the rentals that substitute or delay the question—where a life such as his can go in America.

Prom night, graduation night, too much beer and the radio loud as a banshee. You all but heard the jazzy roadster screech to a halt. Dead end, wreckage.

He pounced on one photo and looked up; 'The future mine! New York.'

He passed it to me; the first prize life bestowed on him, maybe the only one; the apartment where we sat.

'So I came to New York. Some old guy, the friend of a friend, said this place was on the market. The late Seventies. I think he was after my ass; there was quite a session of grab and grope when I came to look at the place. I ran out, said something through the door; to the effect that yes I was interested. In the apartment only, you understand.'

Thus the first inning of the byzantine New York game.

'A message came one day, the old guy says to tell you the apartment is yers. So I started to move in. And the word in the building, as I shortly heard, was: the landlord's dead.

'Strange, he was living in this very apartment, he had some other place in mind for me. And then I got to live in the place where he lived and died. Call it luck.'

No, call it New York.

. . .

Now he spends almost the whole day in bed. He has the telltale look, you can't miss it; sunken eyes, white lips, loss of weight, cadaverous guise.

One day I brought along a container of clam chowder. He sat there on the bed, trying his best to eat; a losing game, he gave up halfway through.

Talk; along these lines. What gave life meaning; 'something more let me tell you than breathing in breathing out'—(especially toward the end, I thought to myself, when in and out are pretty much coinciding).

His younger days, and the proffers that had come his way, this and that—and now and then a gold rush. Seems there was a young lady in his town, quite amenable to the attentions of several suitors—in the direction of board, bed, and beyond. Peter was one of the guests at the communal feast. Seems that at some point, the young woman turned up pregnant.

Then woe and behold. An aunt he described as a Tiger Lady, frowning portentously, showed up at his student dwelling, the messenger of not good news. Seems he was chosen; winner in an open field of candidates. The prize? Why, the hand of the beauty, and more!

Implied strongly, all but stated, was the following. Agreement on his part would issue in transference of (very) large properties and holdings to himself.

But the groom to be—he was not to be.

'No go. She didn't love me, nor I her.'

'More, I knew at the time that I was gay, and that would soon have to be faced.'

He spoke of 'personal success versus making it big in public.' I wasn't persuaded by the choice of words, but they seemed to conceal a truth of moment for both of us.

. . .

The aforesaid led into my story.

Especially the famous eviction from the country in '65.

. . .

I told how a writer showed up at my door lately, wanting a sort of recap of those years, that event. Especially with this query in mind; why did I stick with the Jesuits, given that awful time and its multiple malfeasances—given the fact that so many, who'd suffered far less grievances, had walked away?

The visitor was, if anything, persistent. And I sensed the usual media hype (anything but anything to concoct a headline), something new, something that hadn't been 'covered.'

Peter interrupted. It was a matter, he averred, of playing a game vs. playing your part in life itself. 'In my home town they'd always allow, with a wink, well, Peter is, you know, a bit off the wall, but he's also a good ol' boy. An' wot the hell.

He's gay, we know it, but let's both sides play it, he has the good grace not to rub it in.'

But he did.

'I went back home with Pierre. They could tell, across the wire, what I thought of him, that we were lovers. Though I never used the language, never used even the body language.

'We just were . . . ourselves. An' they knew, an' they put up with it.

'But you understand, I could never go back there, sick as I am with AIDS, and say, Well what do you have to say now? Here I am dyin'. I couldn't do that.'

How alike we were, I thought, in spite of all. How alike in what we had come through.

'Some of 'em would say, what a wasted life, what he could've made of it! But that isn't my feeling about it at all, it's come down to something like, what I've tried to do for others who were in my shoes, what I did for Pierre. I truly believe it—anyone who hasn't wakened to love, hasn't been alive at all.'

On that, he was emphatic as a driven nail. He sat there between smokes, between catches of breath. His eyes were enormous and sunken. Now they no longer simply regarded things, they collided with the world, they all but shot sparks. A slight beard darkened his pallor, the flesh clung to his cheek bones.

Good God, I thought, he's growing into himself, that face we come to deserve—or to be cursed with.

A face, a kind of just deserts. He was resembling, more and more, Saint Sebastian at the stake.

. . .

I went on; my story, oft told, even unto ennui. How I've spoken up, and acted up, and been shipped out or otherwise dealt with.

It seemed to have something to do with his story.

Which, it turned out, included me.

'Oh I see you all right' (rubbing his distended belly). 'You're sure not first of all a priest, or even a Catholic. I say to myself he's just a friend; and leave it at that.'

'What it means, a friend, here's someone sees things along the line I see them. I'm sick, and he keeps coming by. That's all, I don't think of you, priest, Catholic.'

'I'm in trouble, and here he is. That's enough.'

'Everything else's a fraud—they call it making it in public. Jesuit or not, Reagan, religious, it's all the same. They want what America's got to offer.'

He was clear as a bell of passing.

I thought of Turner's ecstatic paintings, all shafts of light, furious and soft and bearing all before, as though creation's splendor and scope poured from simple elemental light, from sky. And then a ship, rich, proud, glistening, making its watery way—toward pure light, its harbor and port of call.

. . .

It was late autumn, winnowing, meager light, days all the more precious for their waning, the sun's largehanded offerings gone, nature on the dole.

He was dying, all the more manifestly as the light failed us. We must read again, and closely, and pay for the lesson, 'The night comes, when no one may work.' And again, 'Come quickly, come Lord Jesus.'

. . .

The summer closed its white-hot hatches. There were pieties in the air.

He was making a good ending. But the images, words, that helped others cope with his passing, were not of his choosing. He clung fiercely to his own resources—the sanity and common sense that had served him well. He simply stood there, or lay there, planted in this world, native to it, the good times and bad passing through his lax hands like two streams.

His years were ample and favoring, meager and thin, like the grainy rings that mark the years in a withstanding tree.

. . .

There was a biblical tone as well. He was not overtly of the prophets, he would make no such claim; religion had served him badly. His life was more like a plod. His mind clung to a beaten path. One step after another; truth assembling itself, subject, predicate, verb, the way to live was revealed piecemeal. Take one step, another opens. Modest, modest—this was the way to proceed in the world.

Indeed there might be a God. The very tentativeness of the assertion stamped it as authentic.

That 'maybe.' It meant that one disdained yapping away, God talk sliding off the tongue, off and out, easy come, quick gone on the vagrant wind.

Vanity of vanities, all is vanity, and indeed and again verily.

And, the eye is not satisfied with seeing, nor the ear with hearing.

And again, there is no remembrance of former things. Nor will there be remembrance of things yet to happen, among those who come after.

. . .

Now his mind was bent, like a bough under snow, toward an improbable bloom, dangerous and unseasonable.

Which is to say, he was incurably hopeful; a very addict of hope. It was another form of his moral strength. He stood free, and he stood with others; so he could be lucid in calling the score, in both directions.

And perhaps the two were one; as though a single bole rising, branched in two, and the two heights took on both task and glory, support and stress.

I marveled. A kind of slovenly hangdog despair would be so easily pardoned him.

But no resigner he. The hope beat its way, on and up.

This is what I remember, what I thank him for. For a cache of gold in a place of ghosts.

Of his hope, there were many beneficiaries. He gave gold away.

· · ·

I had been out of town. A minister phoned; it was his own story he wanted to dwell on, but Peter's as well. That genius of his, that compassionate intervention. The Reverend had been near the end of a frayed rope, ousted from his job, disgraced for the crime of gayness.

Then Peter intervened. I had no details, required none. The minister's tears said it all. Peter had seen him 'through a terrible episode, he had been all heart.'

Yet in Peter's life, recent events had spelled only loss.

He talked laconically of the death of his lover, whom he had cared for to the end; those terrible months. Yes he had lost it all; and no, he was not stymied. While life remained (at least his life), there was a price to pay; for life rightly understood was a kind of pay-as-you-go trip. The planet required fuel, you were aboard. Therefore you paid up.

Let me venture this. Peter, by reason of his persistent, single-eyed love of others, to the disregard of his own sorrowful condition, beyond doubt will attain the vision of God.

. . .

The doctor, young and quite at sea, wonders what to make of this forthright patient, who wants the truth told of his condition. And for the short haul—a milkshake; 'Just to be able to taste . . . something, for God's sake.' The doctor shuffles his papers.

I go out for a milkshake.

In the hospital he was noncommittal, for the most part. For the lesser part he was attentive to the doctors, respectful, but his own man. Who was dying, anyway? Not they, for sure.

The medicos loved him as we did, and mourned the relentless tide, bearing a solitary voyager out and beyond their skills, even beyond their despair.

One said; 'I don't think he's ready to go yet.'

I thought likewise, but it was a help to have her sober, affectionate estimate. More time, we thought, he wants more time. And we were right.

. . .

An ominous message reached me. Posthaste I went to St. Vincent's and his room. He was struggling for breath, an awful hiccupping tearing him apart.

He wanted to go home, that was the burden of his cries, punctuated by the dreadful diaphragmatic staccatos.

'Want to live for a while where I belong, where I can be . . . myself. Can't you help?'

Doctor avers he can, and departs.

And on the instant—here comes old Ecclesiastes again. He looked straight at me. It's like that third eye midforehead of the Buddha. As though in Peter's skull, the other lamps we call eyes, have gone down and down; dim, then hardly a glim. But that third one, how piercing!

'It's all the things those doctors don't say, don't dare say, are important,' he murmurs.

. . .

Another night, then another day. More depleted, less able to cope as dawn comes up.

And an announcement, somewhat depleting in its own right; 'My mother's comin'.'

Now of this ancestor, I've heard something before. On a prior visit from Florida, she lingered amid his febricity less than twenty-four hours. The quick departure seemed, even in the annals of those who find the natives relatively insupportable,—well, hasty. And here, as Peter announces from his pallet resignedly, she comes again.

Here indeed, she indeed.

There is another twist. Mother's motives are, as we used to say, impure. She is a great one for going through properties of son, making hay of what she comes on. 'She arrived here towing this empty suitcase, what she left with I leave to your imagining.'

I await this portent. I am assured that she, daughter of southern Florida waters, desires to meet me.

So we'll see.

He suddenly sits up in the bed, vomiting.

• • •

Much have I traveled in the realms of gold. The realms of terror also, the realms of 'almost' and 'just as good,' realms of very big and of purportedly holy—and all so cruel.

And now, these realms of heroism.

He lay there, pale as a spring bloom daring the deep freeze. He held my hand, wonderingly, as though he was first discovering it, this appendage. 'How tan you are, and look at me, white as death.' As indeed he was.

The talk was about his mother and sundry relatives; they were gathering, Florida to Massachusetts. 'Mama, she wanted to know is this the end, afore she'd invest in an airline ticket. Years ago I would'a said, well, come if you're so minded. This time I said; well, you'd better get your sweet self up here; yes, it's the end all right.'

Thus the bracing converse in a not so loving clan.

All manner of second thoughts are racing about in his fevered head. But this matrilinear visitation awaits a future report.

• • •

One day Peter and I are favored with an astonishing ingress of immaculate cotton coats. In they come! The costumes, tending toward the austere, signify, as we have often been told, a team of healers, skilled, compassionate, available at need.

Five, count them. To ourselves, trembling visitants at a suffering bedside, the descent was formidable, awesome. Five white coats buzz in, armed with the inevitable clipboards and pens, snappy as five flags in a stiff breeze.

The leader stood, as they say, out. He towered, physically, his voice shook the steel rafters, if any. Upon him hands had lain, his was the sinaitic pronouncement—what was going on here? Not to mention, what's to be done about it?

Other doctors in the entourage? They were putty under his thumb, they were dillars and dollars, ten o'clock scholars.

Did they not come and go at other times, singly and in clots, announcing their own evangel, their considered view of the case, issuing instructions, bespeaking their friendship with the sufferer? The hierophant swept them aside.

His concerns were, so to speak, topological. If not ecological.

At one point, he averred that the heat in the room was excessive. As indeed it was. (He was invariably right, it was his illness.) 'Let me show you,' he intoned, suddenly transformed, white coat and all, to a kind of heliolator. As anyone knows, the thermostat can be adjusted. Like this.

He jostled minor characters like myself out of the way, moved to the window, turned a knob or two right or left in the heating unit. Announcement. 'That'll do it.' And departed the precincts, his team of learners and listeners swimming after like a school of guppies.

We were left spinning in his wake, in the wake of his skills, of his arrogance. Quite a specimen.

I learned also the family name, which was a distinguished one, if one is inclined to pay homage to the spectacular international piracies of certain American hegemonies. In Latin America, his clan would be named, in execration or awe, a northern oligarchy.

The New York Jesuits are also linked to his family, as are other Catholic entities, beneficiaries of the piratical mode.

I was much relieved; he gave me not a second glance.

. . .

We plod in and out, out and in, for a period of two terrible weeks, hospital, hospital.

He languishes there, at this writing. Up and down go the fever and ice of mood, up and down the chance and mischance of healing, far and near the hovering of the shadowy interloper. We do not know, no one knows.

Mysterious colorless liquids drip into him, night and day through a maze of intricate tubing. The tubes loop and snake about and make junctures and mix their purported ameliorants and finally dispense them under his skin. It is like a laboratory mockup of the arterial system.

Something too, I mused, of the occult goings-on of a Faustus, in contravention of the noiseless footfalls of death—the approach and kiss of the specter who, until our own lifetime, simply was wont to lay his claim and end things.

They are keeping him alive, but at a price. Death can be bribed, cajoled, made to hang around, wait his turn, like any minor mendicant on the make. What is granted by him to such as Peter (the palm of death being crossed by a number of coins—all those specialists in bribery!) is a kind of twilight zone, a meantime, an existence hardly here, not yet there.

He lingers in that uneasy zone, a character in search of—what? An author? A world?

. . .

Will he die, will he live? Is he doomed here and now? Or will he by hook or crook, medicament or magic, make his way back to what we are pleased to call, knowing no better, 'life today'?

He sits up as though driven by a spasm, cries out, 'O God help me, help me!' His arms thrash about in the air, semaphores signaling to thin air his utmost grief.

He defecates thinly on his sheets. 'The humiliation of the flesh is ours.'

We flash the distress signal over his bed. Some fifteen minutes pass, no one appears. It is the weekend; a skeleton crew, so to speak, of aides and nurses, overworked and harassed, are on duty. Elsewhere.

We take matters in hand. One of our crew goes to the hallway, returns with fresh sheets, purloined.

Clean sheets are spread, Peter is cleansed.

. . .

The mother is in attendance. So to speak.

She views the proceedings stoically from her chair.

Stoicism, or lumpishness, or frostiness, or all three in uneasy confluence—these are her engaging qualities. A faint aura of disgust lies on her face like smudged makeup, a giveaway of the soul's grimace. It turns the corners of her mouth sourly down; her eyes are gelid.

Why has she come? No one can rightly say. From his infancy, she wanted nothing of Peter. Gave him away, as one gives away something used up, or faintly annoying in its needs, or of little value in any case.

Yet the giveaway, appalling as it was, proved providential. He landed with the tenderest of grandmothers.

And now this portent appears in our midst, dethroned but by no means defeated. She stifles our spontaneity, her look strikes us dumb, forestalls the gestures of love we yearn to convey to the sick man.

At some point, her nose quite out of joint, she said to Cary words like these: The scene is physically revolting.

She meant, of course, the sight of shit, and the required bathing of the helpless man.

Cary yielded nothing: If one has the least compassion, he would take up the shit in his bare hands and dispose of it.

. . .

I said farewell to her later. She fixed me with her lidded basilisk gaze, all but impenetrable. 'Take care of his spirit,' she intoned in a voice whose timbre barely attained sea level. Not knowing what it meant, this sudden spurious eruption of spiritual concern, I fled.

One could ponder, long and hard, the needs of her own spirit, as it contrasted with the strength and endurance of his.

Shit no, spirit yes. O gnostic dame!

'Seeing the sick endears them, us it endears too ...
Impatient he cursed at first ...
Child, Felix, poor Felix Randall ...
How far then from forethought of all thy more boisterous years. . . . '

. . .

Have we been through the worst of the current storm? There is no way of knowing. At least the mother has gone on her way. And we are left disconsolate in her wake, to repair the damage as best we might.

Peter looks at me; the look conveys it all. The weekend has been a disaster in nature. And what are we to do, he or I or the Creator of all?

A weekend to be consigned to purgatorial memory. Not merely the visitation of the awful parent. The dearth of nursing and medical attention. None of the staff available, to assuage, to effect some new treatment or continue an old.

. . .

Stymied one day, unable to gain attention, Peter phones someone known in the hospital handbook as a 'patient representative.' Who shortly presents herself. An elderly nun stands before us, four-square from veil to shoon. In pose she is ill at ease, as to powers undefined.

Indeed if power is a synonym for the nudging of an immovable object—it is immediately clear; nothing of the sort is within her ambit.

Peter regards her, eye to eye. He speaks from his diurnal dung heap of his needs and lacks and the long deficiencies of presumably normal service, presumably available.

Why are they not available? Answer me!

She has nothing to say. Noncommittal, a vaporous half-fearful mumbling, then silence.

Yet he is trying with all his might not to be burdensome.

. . .

Willy-nilly, we've started to compose, better, to improvise, a swan song.

Peter's swan song. And ours too; we snatch at the theme with a primordial jealousy. Mine, mine too. But it's a star turn, his only.

In his travail of spirit and body, he hums an anthem common to all.

Listen! So long, so long.

He sighed to me, when I bent over the bed, 'I'm so tired, I don't think I'll make it this time.'

Which he indeed is, which he alas won't.

And again, ever so faintly: 'I didn't think it was going to happen so quick.'

Why we mourn, why we hang around.

Cary has draped a rosary above the bed.

. . .

And here comes a procession we've seen before. They could be (and manifestly are not) morticians, or hired mourners, or knackers, or whoever. Clipboards firmly under arm, all that medical savvy tucked away in the skull.

Immaculately conceived coveralls, earnest, good willed; from furrowed brows, as from the forehead of Jove, issue learned questions, observations, nods, sightings, prognostications.

Never mind that the patient is withdrawn, dying, beseeching only, could they read his tormented eyes, to be left in peace.

'Well, how are you feeling this morning, kindly describe your latest bowel movement, heart movement, head movement.' Notes are taken, heads nod knowingly.

Then, inevitably: 'We're shortly going to do a few more tests' (yet more tests, they'll shortly be testing the meat of a cadaver, but don't worry) 'which it is hoped will reveal etc. etc. and render yourself disposed to keeping on keeping on, less horsepower of course' (no food, no shit, short breath, brain going, heart barely going)—

'—and now if you'll just flip over bunside up, right here'n now we'll do something tried and true, believe you us, the nature of which we can't at present reveal, but which you may be sure will altogether accrue to the benefit of mortal flesh.'

'And those in attendance hereabouts, ever so kindly get yourselves lost, as this blessedly beneficient procedure is about to start. Known as it is only to a few initiates, is, as goes without saying, not for uncircumcised eyes to dwell upon. IF you please.'

Truly a hell of a fix. He's asked only to be kept reasonably comfortable; and here they come sticking him with needles the size of Grandma's darning lances. Till Gawd help us, he resembles Grandma's old-time frayed pincushion. And for what cause, maybe God's privy to, not us.

A mutual rolling of the eyes, his and ours. But we, being obedient if not abject, get ourselves beyond the pale, quick as ink.

. . .

He whispered to me, 'Soon.'

An utterance, by no means opaque, signaling on the part of one lingering for a backward look this side of the pearly portals; Enough, pal. Gawd's sake, let's go.

Is he asking a permission of sorts?

I feel like the warden of a public park, and he, as the Irish say, short taken. What do you do, you let the poor bloke in. So it's after hours, wot the hell. Give 'im a relieving few minutes. And let the law go scratch itself.

. . .

He's coming into possession, ever so slowly and only in part—some inheritance beyond his ken and ours.

It's hovering in the air; Presence, dawn, epiphany.

. . .

Up and down the moods swing.

As whose wouldn't? Up and down, one day and the next, he wants to fight it, he wants to go. One day there's infinite weariness, clouded eye, rasping croak; I've had enough.

I gather courage, tell him in his ear, Peter, let go when you will, don't try so hard, enough is enough.

Another day, in midst of choking and sputtering and mucus unending: I'm still going to fight it.

. . .

I wrote a poem once, and sent it into a jail where Philip was being held. It's entitled 'POVERTY'. Maybe it's about Peter too, I think so:

A prisoner is very poor
1 face, 2 arms, 2 hands
1 nose, 1 mouth
also 3 walls
1 ceiling
10 or 12 iron bars—
then if lucky
1 tree
making it, making it
in hell's dry season
I almost forgot—
No legs!
Contraband! seized!
they stand stock still
in the warden's closet
There
like buried eyes
they await the world

. . .

He lets me bathe his face with cold water. I say, only half in jest, Every day you look more like Christ. First thing you know, they're going to be coming in here with lit candles, make an ikon of you.

He cracks a rare smile.

. . .

Voice all but gone, he puts matters simply, with hand signals; 'The hardest thing of all, not being able to talk.'

. . .

One day I told him, I'd be out for the evening, a poetry reading on Park Avenue, of all places. I'd do my best to see him afterward. He croaked; Well, I'll sure be here, I ain't going nowhere.

. . .

What to make of this.

He's coming back. From the hell of the past four weeks. From intestinal cancer, from fevers and chills, from two weeks of tubes in nose and throat, from ... death's open door.

He's eating again, his thin hands stretch out in greeting, the bones of a small bird, all atremble with weariness and weakness. As though he's asking wordlessly, am I still here? Or there? Or where?

The enormous eyes focus with difficulty, he turns to the attendant, guest, those he loves, those he bears with—slowly, with enormous effort.

He's like a foundling, rescued against all hazard, brought indoors by loving hands. Unable to believe his good fortune; too sudden, too dear.

And his good luck is ours. The doctors bustle about, proud as new parents. He's made it back!

We don't know for how long, no one does. Long or short, it's no more than a respite.

. . .

Behold, I reflect in a quiet moment, this one. Who in easier time instructed us sternly; no more chemo, no more tubes, supplements, antibiotics; No mas, dammit!

And then a sea change. He reached a new resolve, somewhere in the dark that lies behind the eyes. Words he had spoken, instructions issued in comparative ease and health—these were invalidated. He resolved to live.

The images that govern dying were radically altered. Other images, of life, combat, patience, courage, took hold.

. . .

I had urged; Go when you want to.

He listened intently, but in his soul he said no. Or so I reconstruct things. Going with the tide, the current, easing out—the images were too facile; they failed to befit the strict cut of his will. The presumed—neutral weather, a tepid sea. He would have none of it.

So he tacked, cut sideways, headed straight into the wind. He would change course, at all cost. And if he sank, that too was part of the risk. Implicit in the bargain his champion's heart made with . . . Someone.

I never promised you a Dead Sea.

. . .

It was the eve of Thanksgiving. I brought him red roses, five of them.

I chose the flowers like a gourmet, one by one.

Arrived in his room.

The bed was empty.

I knew a brief moment of panic. In such a world as we daily walk, any conceivable catastrophe is possible. Either he had died as many AIDS patients go, like the careless dropping of a second shoe—or he had been discharged, gone home.

My roses and I, each paled by a terrible prospect, sought out a nurse.

Home he had gone, within hours. 'And not in the best of spirits,' she sniffed, as though four tormenting weeks and spotty hospital care should have sent him off with a hoarse huzzah! Come now. I had wit enough to thank her fervently for 'all you've done for him.'

Done for him, done to him? The compliment was puffed by relief, and two-edged at that. She was by no means one of the worst of his recent afflictions.

I phoned, Cary answered, jubilant. 'Yes, Daniel, he's here all right, sitting up. Weak, though.'

. . .

One day in the hospital phase, Cary and I were taking a lunch break from our vigil. He referred longingly to a trip he planned, 'to see my grandmother in California.' 'And when?' I asked. 'Oh, post-Peter.'

We all know what is coming—and it matters not a whit.

There is the gift of the hour, to be revelled in, to set the heart dancing.

. . .

Are we prepared for life? We shall see. But for now, to live is . . . anything but a task. A celebration. 'It is fitting to make merry and be glad; for this your brother was dead, and is alive; he was lost, and is found.' Viva Peter.

. . .

For awhile; everything for awhile.

He returned home; his condition improved no whit.

Then we were back in the terrors of five weeks ago.

They went like this, the intractable latter days. I would appear in his room, to no perceptible welcome. He lay there, turned to the wall. Grouchy, cross grained, most unlike.

'It's do this for me, hand me that, and at all hours,' Cary mourned, nearly at wits' end.

We enlisted Kathy the nurse, no novice in difficult matters.

'It's just that he's dying,' she ruminated, 'and of course it's tough having healthy people hopping in and out. I've often seen how depression sets in when people return home after a long stay in hospital. Life has been so organized, all sorts of people coming and going. And don't forget, there's no magical return to health just because he came home. . . . '

One thing grows clearer; it's our dark night as well as Peter's.

. . .

It was the first Sunday of Advent. We Christians are counseled by the liturgy of the season to wait, to be alert, to attend even 'sleeplessly,' a mysterious event referred to as 'the coming of the Lord.'

It is no infantile message. Inserted in the gospel of this day are unsettling images of catastrophe and horror and loss. Preludes, we are told, to another event, to occur 'in this generation.'

. . .

I take the Peter event, and its repercussions on us, as a hint of this 'prelude.' Like those awaiting we know not what, we sit in darkness and sorrow, sensing that something portends, Someone awaits.

We wait there, cling to the sick man. For the most part we are in the dark. The 'signs' are mysterious, awesome.

We have inklings. But we are far from faith.

We spread out the pitiful flea market of our souls, keep vigil there, knowing our condition, our need. Saying nothing.

Then the curtain rises.

Something takes form, stupendous and sweetly familiar at once.

And imagine, we are invited.

We cannot imagine, even when a new world, new heavens and earth, are being unveiled (seven veils) before us.

The dying of Peter.

Dying yes, death no. What the Irish refer to as a 'hard dying.' There are crises, seeming points of no return. And he does not die. He clings there for all of autumn, into Advent, Christmas nearing. And he speaks, when he can speak at all, in a hoarse whisper, of 'going home for Christmas.'

He's not waxing pious, be it added in haste.

'If I go home for Christmas, I want assurance my room here'll be kept for me.' We nod, we'll try our best; at this point we'd agree to anything.

. . .

I was down and out with a wicked cold. And averred to the nun that I'd best not visit the sick man, for fear of infecting him with yet another woe. She was brisk, even starchy, waved my objection aside. 'No, go and see him. He's been asking for you. And what difference can anything make at this point?'

So I went. He was functioning strictly on borrowed time. The borrowing had gotten positively larcenous; whoever was the lender couldn't win.

How repay? Out of what capital?

. . .

Indeed I wondered. Do there exist somewhere, beyond our ken, in a kind of spiritual Fort Knox, great golden ingots of time, proof against all careless or covetous transactions in the world? That world where, it is said, people waste time, give time, buy time, do hard time (jails) or easy. The world where, moreover, a type invariably named Scrooge grinds his molars in the night, convinced beyond argument that time is money. And in pursuit of each, accumulates vast stores of both.

. . .

Peter has a teaching to offer, concerning time, its coming and fleeing. We mortals must operate, it would seem, on a larger scale of time than the next breath or heartbeat. Indeed we are by nature very spendthrifts of time; which is to say, we fancy ourselves thrifty, in the act of spending. We use time somewhat as we use the Earth, as though time were eternal, and the Earth boundless. To our dismay we are learning otherwise.

. . .

For Peter (no Scrooge he) time was running out; the ingots, the minutes, were melting, falling away in the furnace of mortality.

Sister said, 'He nearly went a week ago. I gave him, say, twelve hours. And the next morning, can you believe, he was sitting up eating breakfast.'

He fades hourly from the expectation of the living, falls away from his own living resemblance; that image we carry of him, the one we lived by and loved.

The metamorphosis comes and goes. Much depends on the drugs they're pumping into him on whatever day. Some days he puts on what Cary calls his 'owl eyes and shaking hands.' Like a shaman bird costume, worn for a sacred passage. And then in an onset of ecstatic seizure, form and function marry, the costume becomes . . . the person.

. . .

Humor saves a day—or at least an hour. Cary announced, as some friend's proposal, that when we eventually dispose of Peter's and Pierre's remains, we also include the ashes of their dog, recently translated to the great canine mansion in the sky. I'm not sure the rather winsome, bizarre suggestion will win Peter's OK. Nor can one predict the ideal occasion on which to broach the subject of this proposed doggy apotheosis. We shall see.

. . .

Down with a stubborn flu, I wince and groan and send a prayer southward. How fares Peter?

. . .

Finally toward morning, the coldest of the year; phone rings at 3:10 AM. My prophetic bones.
It is Cary, and his news. 'The great man is gone. Died peacefully.'

. . .

There was talk, weeks later, of assigning me another patient, and who it might be.

'You understand,' one of the nurses said gamely, 'there won't be another Peter, they don't come twice.'

The grammar was wobbly, the point clear. As if I needed telling.

. . .

On a peerless July afternoon, in the Atlantic ocean off Block Island, we performed the final pieties by scattering Peter's ashes.

The borrowed sailboat and its crew leapt clear of land with a celerity that seemed, to amateur eyes, the blur of a thoroughbred drinking the wind.

We read first from the burial service of the dead at sea: 'Unto God we commend the soul of our brother departed. And we commit his body to the deep in sure and certain hope of the resurrection unto eternal life, through our Lord Jesus Christ ... at whose coming ... to judge the world, the sea shall give up its dead. And the corruptible bodies of those who sleep in Him shall be changed and made to resemble His glorious body. . . . '

From the Gospel of John: 'Jesus said, "Let not your hearts be troubled; you believe in God, believe also in me. In my Father's house there are many mansions. I go to prepare a place for you. And I will come again, and receive you to myself. . . . " '

And finally from Revelation: 'Then I saw a new heaven and a new earth ... God will dwell with God's people, ... will wipe every tear from their eyes. And death shall be no more, neither shall there be mourning nor weeping, for the former things have passed away. . . . '

The moment came, the boat (or was it ourselves?) shivered as we sped. Months of waiting, years of travail, all ended. We took in hand the sack of human ash, the small light residue of one we loved and wept for. All gone in flame, all but Peter's spirit, whose agile symbol and new element were the racing prow and the living waters that sped us along.

The boat leaned gently, as though a providence held us in its palm. The ashes fell and fell. They met the waters in a scaly cloud and sank on the instant. No trace, no wake, Peter's name written in water.

It was simple, easeful, final, after the ferocious ice and fevers of life. Each of us took up a handful of wild blossoms, and tossed them after. The flowers rode the waves lightly, a wake of memory.

SIX

THE TIME TOLD AWRY, THE TIME TOLD RIGHT

*That face which is not my own
and my own
—that death which is not my own
and my own*

M eeting Richard for the first time; another ingredient of the sorrow of this endless summer, one torrid day sliding into another, fire meeting fire, raging by day, banked by night, little or no respite. After awhile, we're convinced that 'this is the way things should be, therefore they are,' a procrustean principle, and unconsoling. Necessity becomes law; we languish in a very kingdom of necessity.

. . .

And what, in such a horrid instance, would the king of necessity look like?
We have some inkling at least. Under the guise of death and hell lurks, more or less concealed, the face of the one who would rule over such existences as ours.
The kingdom would resemble the 'justice system,' I reflect, after a visit to my brother Phil in the slammer in Virginia. The world as slammer; eye for an eye, death for death, everyone condemned to an equivalent iron-walled last mile, a world as defined and regulated and architecturally apt as a death row.
Oh, to be in charge of a world like that! What a vindication of one's sour smoldering quarrel with existence itself! And no

quarrel with the ruinous unmaker of lives; lives that finally, in the mind of the king of necessity, are 'of no worth.'

. . .

Summer, Philip in jail, shunted about from one county to another. For a time no one knows where he is, letters are returned, he disappears in the maw of the system.

Meantime, the quadrennial clown school plays in New Orleans; the Republican conventicle simmers away in the ruinous season, something between a theater of cruelty and absurdity. Miles of smiles, all that money, all that huffing and puffing, the lies, the promises-promises, the shouting, the drunks tottering about witless, the klieg lights that strike one blind....

. . .

We are being instructed, in a thousand foul ways, how to 'make it.' At whose expense is of little matter, nor the cost paid—those who pay being others than ourselves, the place of payment invariably elsewhere.

Still the cost is never canceled. Those who pay lurk like uneasy ghosts in the shadows cast by the great orb of Gog in New Orleans. They pay and pay: the homeless in our streets, the peasants of Nicaragua.

. . .

I want to learn (and I don't want to learn) the opposite; how to lose. As others are losing, well and nobly.

May one thus unlearn, gradually, the lessons of the culture? Lessons which, all said, come down to a simple calculus: how to win, and the devil take the hindmost.

. . .

Every Titanic sinks. There was, they boasted, only one. And it refused to coexist with the seas, to reverence the might of another, far greater power. It must win. Therefore it lost.

Do we, like ships too proud, too weighty, sail off and simply go under, as sign that creation cannot bear the weight, the pride? If this were all, what interest would attach to death— or indeed to life itself?

. . .

The great spirits of our species are a vindication, a 'something more,' they are worth watching. They bring drama and a great cry, to the inevitable. Thereby transforming it to . . . vocation, choice, celebration.

. . .

I want to learn something, to lose and gain something. Else why set out time and again, on another of these quests; for friendship or hope or a turn of the road, and what (or who) waits beyond.

By way of pointing me on my way, there is the usual meager description supplied by one of the nurses; so-and-so would love to meet you, I'm sure you would get along quite well. . . .

Which, as to the latter speculation, invariably comes true, shortly and quite wonderfully.

From northwest Manhattan, I make my lurching way south, then east. And land on Main Street, Funkyville, USA. A recognition flashes; within the week, inflamed by torrid weather and egged on by the taunts of residents and others, the cops have run amok along this same pavement. They chased and wounded anyone at hand—strollers on the street, those taking late air on stoops, those peaceably returning home. No one's errand or credential exempted him from the blows of the black and blue brigade. Into Thompkins Square they poured, the victims running before; a sorry summer night, and the law 'n' order boys giving chase.

. . .

I come on the house, ring the bell and wait. My man appears to say his feeble welcome and ushers me indoors.

What had once been a substantial human frame wavers there in the doorway, cadaverous, a Van Gogh skull, eyes blazing away like a concentrate of noon.

We enter a tiny apartment commonly known as a 'railroad flat.' Windows front and rear, other divisions of rooms quite arbitrary; alcoves succeed one another, borrowing whatever dignity from species of mullioned overhang, change of colors, suggestions of passage. The rear and front exposures offer the only daylight; moons, so to speak, to a common sun.

. . .

The forty-day heat spell had partially broken; the day was bearable. I had planned, tentatively, a venture into the neighborhood for coffee. But Rick had his own ideas, and a cold drink appeared. So we sat, and sized one another up.

What he saw I leave to the recording spirits, hoping the quill is dipped in sweet charity.

What I saw was a slow-moving angular figure of forty years or so, peremptorily cut to more modest size than the earlier pattern indicated. Snip, snip had gone the scissors; and presto! the customer bore the lean look of one being fitted, rapidly or slowly, for a final costume.

The emotional tone aroused in this preliminary viewing (in course of which one discerns a temporary version of the final product, pinned and tucked up and marked for hemming and stitching by the fine hand of the master tailor, the choice of material and style and heft and weave being not the customer's but snootily his alone)—nevertheless, and all this taken in consideration, the tone of the meeting is . . . serenity.

A serenity worthy the marmoreal.

Marmoreal? Discard the metaphor. His serenity sits like the finest mesh, a cloud of cobweb descends on the bone and flesh of the living.

A claim? The word is too harsh to be borne, too close.

Serenity sits on him like a stigma; more than a claim, the acceptance of the claim.

Come in. A word spoken to someone else than me, someone who has slipped in, all unannounced, before me.

. . .

Conjure us then, seated opposite one another in that tiny cell sipping our tea like two gentlemen of Verona or Penzance—or Nirvana. Practitioners of an art or two; call it prestidigitation or saving fiction. Call it the art of living.

We agree to make the occasion, a meeting of two strangers, a consequent stillness—to make of these elements, in word and wordlessness—a rebuke, a setback offered death.

A setback offered the kingdom of necessity, whose implacable governor would, if he dared, blunderbuss his way in, uncontrollable as the true blue street thugs of the past week.

No, he is at bay; he has no say.

We two shall meet for an hour or so, chat quietly, decide where this occasion and its quiet outcome, like twin rivulets slowly converging, shall come together in some larger stream we name future.

Death shall not be a third party to all this. No vote, not even an absentee ballot. Down, dog!

. . .

Rick had been a carpenter and plasterer, until—. It was an old story, but the pain was new, a fresh turn of the blade.

'I have to say no, can't accept work. I remember once agreeing, after my first bout of illness, that I'd plaster the ceilings of a house in Queens. To make matters worse, the elderly couple had moved everything out of their three bedrooms and were in effect making do in kitchen and dining room. I thought I'd have the work done in a matter of four days.

'And then one morning, the morning I was to start, I woke up with a vile fever, hardly able to get to the phone, to say it was all off.

'You see what I mean.'

. . .

He's housed by a friend. The apartment, small enough to afflict a snail with cabin fever, now houses his host and himself.

Two railroaders, willy-nilly, cheek by jowl in a boxcar and caboose!

A magnificent grand piano is one of the unlikely amenities of the front room.

'Andrew's a concert star,' Rick says simply. 'He used to teach piano here in the apartment. Then I got ill. He was with me night and day in the hospital. And when they released me, I had nowhere to go. He took me in. Now he can't bring students in; no room. So he lives off his savings.'

All his sentences are flat, to the point. He launches them on the air in what the old notations of Gregorian chant used to call *tono directo*. Translate: sing it out clear.

It's heartbreaking and noble and all but unheard of in New York. Where grab and run and get what's yours has been elevated to a codicil of the Decalogue.

Take someone into your home? Someone ill unto death, and a death such as even Job on his worst recorded day hadn't imagined?

'He took me home.' I hadn't heard it before, and yet I had. Dorothy Day 'took people home.' In her intemperate and insistent manner, and armed with the credential of someone who had first done what she commended, she declared that parishes and rectories and convents should do likewise.

Some of which did. Most of which did not.

(And let it be added that this Jesuit has not so far done so. And is by no means proud of the confession.)

. . .

I departed, having invited him and his unlordly landlord to sup at my place anon. The following Saturday, for instance? He was delighted, and for his own part accepted.

So we shall see. Where a good start might lead.

. . .

He came as scheduled, braving the heat and subway delays and breakdowns. Looking for all the world like death at the feast; but no death in his blue eyes! Only fair speculation, as he looks you in the face, and the world as well, and finds it (and presumably you) good.

Bearing a bottle of wine in his rucksack, a gift of some note, since like most of the afflicted, he's anything but affluent.

Another AIDS friend, Peter, was in attendance. It was the first time we had under the roof two such ill men, and I was in considerable uncertainty as to how things would go.

How well things went!

This despite the truly awful condition of Peter, barely on his feet, yet staggering uptown; a measure of his high regard for a specimen like me; a measure also, I suppose, of his loneliness.

I'd feared the conversation would get waterlogged with pity or presentiments of disaster or a display of mutual symptoms. They spoke of such matters for awhile, and then gently proceeded toward topics of more communal interest. A generally decent political sense prevailed, easing among other humanities the sense of personal tragedy.

Toward nine o'clock, Peter faded and departed. Rick was much inclined to stay on; for an hour or so he offered details of his life. That he had been for a short time a brother in a religious order, the novitiate situated in the Hudson valley. It developed, moreover, that I had visited the premises in the early Sixties, some time before he entered the community. These were pleasant convergences.

He speaks gently, his manner is shy.

It helped, I think, to jog his mind toward acceptance of a newfound friend, that I had visited him at his home, and left a book, 'Portraits'—'to help you know me,' as I explained.

An artist and poet, God wot. Though I have yet to see his work.

His family, he says, is at his side in his illness and its dire implication. His mother helps finance his precarious existence.

. . .

Sometimes it is as though a pit were opening under my feet.

Or as though creation's innocent face suddenly broke in a sardonic contortion; Come now, let me show you another side of things.

Or as though the apparent solidity of the earth were in fact the frailest of crusts.

It all comes to this, as far as I can understand (not very far!)—One is forbidden to breathe the air of our world, rejoice in its beauty, and all the while remain in ignorance—of despair, delusion, fear and loss. Come down, come down.

I can only respond, with hands empty and outspread—Do with me.

Do as You will with Rick and Peter and so many others, who are dying. And I at their side, helpless. From somewhere, in the bitter meantime, summoning the strength—strength to be helpless, to stand there. And now and again, to offer friendship—a meal, a few hours' surcease. So pitifully little; yet something.

. . .

The bully boys live on, and thrive on their meaty diet of deception and headhunting. And the gentle folk go under. No wonder one of them says something to the effect that 'if there is a God, there's an accounting ahead!'

I look into the gentle tormented face of Rick. Or I visit my brother for a scant hour in the rude den, the jail of Alexandria. And under the elixir of those pure and courageous glances—the ill, the prisoner of conscience—there arises in me like a long-frozen sap, a longing to reverse the very course of the world. Revelation, judgment. To reclaim the lost art of justice, to vindicate the victims, to purge public life, if only for awhile, of its parasites. To turn to nothing the habiliments and styles of power. To reveal the illness that infects the powerful. To summon the perpetrators at long last to an accounting for their crimes.

And then in testimony of another way, to summon the ill, the prisoners, the poor, so patient and gentle in the bearings of their burden. To invite them, unaccustomed as they are, and clumsy as they are bound to be, to their rightful place in the world—the seats of power. With a simple mandate, simply announced; to initiate at last a new order of things.

The gentle and clean of heart, the poor of spirit and rich in grace, the mourners, the peacemakers—to thrust in their hands the reins of the world's course! Summon from the shadows the tortured and disappeared, open the madhouses and jails, let the King of Hearts issue forth, to lead the dance!

We hardly dare imagine this. We hardly can summon to mind what decent political conduct might look like. We see through a dark glass indeed the dim outlines of a just world. We peer like timid savages through the mists of morning; dimly, there appears a clearing in the jungle. Decent folk dwell there; they go serenely about their tasks and joys; living, dancing, begetting, cherishing.

But even as we look, a doubt arises in our hearts; is this a mirage, confabulated out of longing and outrage and nothing more? The mists vanish, the people of the mist along with them. And we sorrowfully turn to the jungle again; our native terrain, wild dog eat dog, the only life (life?) we know.

. . .

And then I pull up in my tracks. The only life? There exists another way. And many are doing their level best to live it, day to day and hour by hour. To live it despite all. Though the way we live and love and work seems to go nowhere in the world, is regarded as arcane, faintly dangerous—in any case quite beside the point; a kind of cottage industry for malcontents, for those incapable of making it, big and loud, according to the common norms of the culture. Norms which in the last awful decade have taken on the aura and substance of a divine approbation.

. . .

America sees us, nonviolent folk, resisters, as something like dwellers in one of those reconstituted villages, costumes and decor, false fronts and dance and labor preordained by some awful Department of National Folklore.

But the real question is other; not how they see us, but how we see ourselves, under God.

. . .

What wild and wonderful imaginings! And all awakened by an evening with two desperately ill men. Also by a visit (if it could be dignified as such), phone in hand, thick plate glass intervening, with my brother in jail.

The chaplain's word came back, when I requested a 'contact visit' with Phil. Talk about scripture dragged murkily to whatever abusive misuse! Said in effect, that 'blood was thicker than spirit, therefore there should be no exception made for two brothers. Request denied.'

As the song has it, ironically, 'And they'll know we are Christians by our love. . . . '

. . .

So we have at hand presently these two: Rick, who has left the church behind; and Peter, who apparently never knew in this department anything more robustiously winning than the Baptist ravings he describes with such ardor—in midthunderation he speedily ran for the hills.

Thank God for Peter and Rick, recently stopping for refreshment in these premises, and blessing me in the doing. So that I felt for a time 'under the shadow of thy wings' in my mortal tent, recalling as I do Abraham's mysterious visitants.

Thus I bear, and Phil can bear, that afflictive spirit referred to above. Religious or secular, one rampage, one fear, one violence.

The hooves thunder toward one, then—then 'horseman pass by.'

. . .

Phil told me of a method he has adopted for coping in jail. Coping in the present instance with four transfers from one pokey to another, with the chains and cuffs, with the unknown destinations and the oh-so-well-known prospects, with the polluted din of the TV tube drumming at one's skull night and day.

Simply, he takes pen and Bible in hand each morning and writes a brief meditation from Luke's gospel. This, he says, is the only way available to him, of praying.

I think these notes are something in the same vein. A way of coping with the world. The world, be it added hastily, as something other than a vivid and breathing artifact and triumph of the living God.

The world as derelict and nearly defunct, an image of the lost street people I encounter daily.

. . .

A tough three weeks, lurching into four. Peter in and out of dying. And then Rick too is back in hospital. So the weary round continues.

I found him in the course of a visit, quite congested; a return of the nemesis, pneumonia. I sat and chatted awhile. Could I bring him anything? Well, maybe a book or two. Of what vintage? Poetry or short stories would be wonderful.

A few days later, he was much improved. Andrew, who has stood by through all this, was present.

. . .

You have it all by heart, you've seen it before. And yet it hurts so in the telling. A friend is down, all but out, then up again briefly. And finally, for him the bell tolls; down for good.

And you—you've been given another, bitter task. You're recording the fall; fall from public grace, from health and family, from attachments that wring the heart even as they are surrendered.

What to do? Only the little that seems, in wintry season, a veritable nothing. And yet that 'little' sounds its penny whistle note in the darkness; an interlude, a relief.

. . .

This dear man; he fades. He dwells at home, compassionately cared for by a friend who confesses to being utterly exhausted. But what's to be done? Rick is not so ill as to require hospitalizing (and who wants that in any case?)—too ill to attempt even to rise from bed.

One day he tried to reach me on the phone. The sound that emerged one would imagine issuing from a talking raven, a high toned croak and no more. I barely made it out. 'Hello there' and so on; and 'I'm so-so,' and so on.

Quoth the raven, he's nearing the end of his sojourn. And mercy would respond mournfully, 'the sooner the better.'

. . .

'No longer are you to be named "Forsaken," nor your land "The Abandoned." ' (Isaiah, 62:3) I thought of this, how we name ourselves to our own soul, often in a way contrary to God's naming of us. 'But you shall be called "My Delight," and your land, "The Wedded One." ' (v. 4) In our deepest heart we name ourselves: Nobody, Nowhere. A matter of depression, of ill will, of dwelling upon ill treatment—by fate or fortune or whatever; there is no end to it.

At the same time, we've deliberately (or perhaps inadvertently) misnamed the world we walk in. 'Desolation, Detour, Lost Garden, No Way, Dead End.' An equal denial. It betrays the Original Naming, which was prior in existence to the disaster we name original sin. First the Naming, then the Misnaming. But first things first.

I bring up such matters, to myself of course—and then thinking of Rick, and his all but nameless going. Unknown to me; or virtually so. He's the first to say farewell without having in any real sense said hello. Shy, rendered doubly withdrawn by his illness, which transforms laughing lallygagging folk all so quickly into a species of crustacean hermits. Some scuttle sidewise away, away, dig themselves a pit. And disappear.

And what are their thoughts, in the course of their subterranean frenzy, such lust for darkness, for final solitude, for 'leave me alone!'? Who can rightly tell? They take thought, they mourn, they rage; then they close off and fall asleep.

And the meaning of it all, as it touches on those they love, is no more than the hum of a shell held to the ear. The lovers and friends, survivors and mourners, take up with a sense of infinite loss and grief all that remains; that shell of a life.

Memories; voices come back, the stuff of memories. The great sounds, the frenzies, Lear on the heath, Job on his offal heap—all who made no peace with iron fate. These are distilled, calmed, melded in one. The hum of a distant sea, or of the dark void between ourselves and the stars.

Or as though ... Someone took this life into altogether loving, tender arms; then hush, oh hush the night cry of a child shaken by its dreams.

. . .

I came too late to become a friend. There was good will on both sides, a good start, a spontaneous generous will to see what might come of this.

Little came of it. He was already on a road he had chosen, his alone.

To make too much of this is to belittle the decision. Which was after all his, by rights. Almost by birthright, at least as he read his rights. Who would accompany him, and how far, and at what pace; and who not.

I tagged along, made calls now and then, listened to the plaints of his friend (night chores, day chores, the long run of the illness). Offered what consolation I could, keeping the offer open, 'to stop by, when you think he'd like a visit.'

Which he seldom did. Until the end.

. . .

There lay the dying man in the parlor. He was stretched under a coverlet, he looked like a St. Francis by Zurbaran, all eyes and pointed beard and burning skull. The cowl was a matter of shadow in the faint light of January evening, a shadow gathering around him as well as ourselves; but ritually and close, around him closest of all. I knelt and greeted him; there was only the faintest of responses; the dying Francis.

His mentor and nurse and friend Andrew ventured out for an hour or two with me, to dine and gain a measure of surcease. Before leaving, we bent over our Francis and informed him of our purpose. The patient nodded faintly, closed his eyes and resumed his dreamy mental plod. Another enterprise than ours lay on his mind.

We settled on a Japanese restaurant in the neighborhood. Andrew was hungrier for talk than for provender. To my questioning, the sense of his answers: 'Rick is a genius, you know, highest intelligence ratings, an artist and poet.'

'As to his family, there are varying Catholic shudders and a measure of plain indifference. Most people find an excuse for walking away, don't they?'

'He's a friend of many years; I should perhaps make it clear'—(there was a sudden vehemence in his voice, he leaned toward me)—'I'm not his lover, you know. Or did you know?'

I didn't know one way or another, and cared less. And said so. He seemed reassured.

'Two years ago, I learned that Rick was in hospital. I visited him; then someone told me, no one wants him, he has nowhere to go. On an impulse I said, let him come to me. I'll take care of him.

'And you understand, I hadn't the slightest notion of what that would involve. I only heard the words, he has no one. And I thought, Yes he does. He has me.'

. . .

Never once have I responded to someone in such a way. (Maybe, once or twice, tried gingerly to walk that thin line.) But to meet someone homeless on the street, saying on impulse, Come home with me. And then to discover the consequence; this someone, this new-found friend is ill, God help us, very ill. And God above all help me; I've taken on a task that may well break my bones.

The facts would be these. For a large slice of my life, this presence will put everything else in question. Career? Leisure? Livelihood even? Go from my hand, sweet birds of youth.

. . .

Such style, this friend of Rick, a very mandarin! That precise voice, soft as cat's feet, that understatement of life's alarms and passages, the suavity, a foil for a gemlike endurance.

His tailoring, like his whole presentment, is impeccable.

One day we sit together in the hospital corridor. Like a blast from Olympus, the raucous summoning system interrupted our talk. Dr. so-and-so is to proceed immediately here or there, the voice pierces to the bone, much like the decibel turnup of a subway announcement or the gabble over airplane loudspeakers. Is the fault bad technology, or are American voices plain ugly?

We talk, and the overblast continues. We raise eyes to the oracular ceiling, read one another's lips and fill in the blanks.

Andrew; an unhappy childhood. Religion; an ingredient of the unhappiness. From age seventeen, on his own. Inability, even today, to connect with his family; especially, and perennially, on the matter of sexuality.

It comes to me, so to speak. He's one of those internal expatriates who by hook and crook make their way to New York, out of one or another form of bondage. A few survive the trek, the shock of landing. Many go under in the welter of the world's biggest flea market; destruction for sale, for barter, for free.

We talk the sun down.

*'In my walks it seems to me
that the grace of God is in courtesy.'*

This Chinese gentleman of an old school! Alas, the masters have fled the premises or died, the building is long closed and boarded up and transmogrified into ... what? A condo cage for outrageous pelts and plumage?

Such lessons as were once considered useful—deportment, courtesy, discipline, the ceremony of tea or flowers, the rhythms of the heavens and seasons, these are no longer offered. The school is closed, the graduates long scattered. They have learned, no doubt, ways of thriving in the world, ways derived from the infinite capacities of the almighty dollar. A code is vanished from the earth. Noblesse oblige? Say rather, ignoblesse.

Noblesse, Andrew. Underscored. The aristocrat knows when a shockeroo is in order, how to send it forth, understated, light as a bird's exhalation. 'I've cleaned shit for awhile,' he smiles, all but purring with subdued oxymoronic humor. It is as though he sedately inhabits a world that is created in his image, elegant, civilized, well ordered. 'That ought to qualify for friendship, hadn't it?'

He rises quickly. 'Can we check on Rick, he may have awakened?'

The patient has, to a degree only. One thinks for a weird moment on entering—a mask, regal, doomed, has been set there in the bed, that and nothing more.

The head rolls about, this way, that, seeking . . . what? The eyes are all but unmoored in their sockets.

We touch hands to his face, the poor lorn buoy grows still for a moment, calm on his miserable sea. A glance comes to rest on Andrew, on me, a question unspoken. As though, God help the helpless, we were some unlikely epiphany of the almighty. Why cannot I die?

The question torments us as well.

. . .

'They alone attain the promised land who know nothing of where they are going.'

This is how he went. One day in late winter, Andrew summoned me, urgently. 'Please come. I must have help. He's been vomiting blood, is quite beside himself.'

Down and across I made my way, through East Fourth to St. Mark's Place, that grand Gogolesque neighborhood, the

East Village. Everything improbable in human life and conduct and costume is there rendered commonplace, rears toward one in stark bold display.

Block after block, they saunter about, preen, couple hands and arms. The store windows are mirrors; are we the living, are the clones there or here? It is as though a coven of mannequins had escaped their fenestrations, and wandered about like the undead, chalky of face, wild of wig; centaurs unhorsed, emblems of a last day, or a history we thought long past.

Long past? Here we are offered on one street sauntering Indian braves, the hair cut like an upstanding mane, and Japanese samurai, livid of grimace, and frontiersmen in their fringed jackets of soft leather. And divas of varied age and tragic mien, their eyes blacked with kohl.

I threaded my way, passed from this vociferous crowd of innocents, these singers of the siren song of no death. And entered the portal of peace and twilight. Our patient was quite visibly dying.

He continued vomiting blood, as we held him, spoke as tenderly as we might of companionship on that bleak last mile of his, and all uphill. His breathing stertorous, he calling out Help me, Help me.

His head tossed witlessly this way and that, his poor sticks of arms made wild gyrations in the air; tracing what? The Presences gathering? The form of things to come? He seemed at times to be beckoning, at others repelling.

One hand was cold to the touch, the other hot. He lay as one who lingered this side and that of the mirror of the world. As though the breath of life were departing, and he half here, half there. The flesh clothed him partially, the permeable spirit was shaking it off, that abused vestment; and time too, leading his poor mortality, so gradually, so tragically, part way.

'We lingered yet by the ocean marge, as they

*who think upon the road that lies before
and in their mind go, but in body stay. . . . '*

Then like Dante's guide through the silva obscura and beyond, we must all glide away. He was going alone.

He was bleeding, he was dehydrated, he seemed also to be choosing. Andrew leaned close, called in his ear; 'Do you want to return to the hospital, Richard?'

The hospital once more? But what benefit could a hospital offer at this dire stage? And could not a catastrophe be precipitated on the way, with the banging and pummeling and lifting up and thumping down? Why not abide in peace, with us?

Go for it. Andrew phoned the police. They arrived as though out of thin air, dispassionate, efficient. 'The ambulance is on the way,' one of them announced. 'We'll wait for it outside.'

A siren sounded, the medics came in jacketed and scarved against the frigid night. 'Seems as though I've been here before,' one of them mused, readying equipment, wasting neither words nor effort.

They uncovered him; then a horror, a stench. Even the medic was shaken. He turned to us. 'Didn't you know he's been bleeding rectally?' Indeed he had bled, a dark infected stain penetrated sheets and mattress.

They bore him out. At the doorway I saw the tormented head fall to one side. The others hardly knew, but I knew.

Andrew followed them, a friend and I stayed, cleaning up as best we might, rolling up sheets and coverlets for burning. We were sobered and silent; the swift assault upon that poor life!

Outside, the medics pursued their crisis routine, hustled his frame into the ambulance. But he was gone, they knew it.

The death was an illustration, a questioning of an ordinary, all but banal occurrence. Who does not, several times each day, go from his house on this or that errand, with full expectation of return?

But that doorway of Andrew's became a kind of classic Greek portal in my mind. He bowed out, like Hecuba or Clytemnestra or Oedipus; in that precinct he grew still, forever.

. . .

Next to his bed hung one of his paintings, it glimmered there in the dark.

He had painted a cool rectangle, a grid of light and dark blue. Here and there along the straight tracks and angles, a bright red square flashed out. It was sophisticated and atavistic at once; spirit, newly released from bondage, emitted tracers of light, as it ventured through a dark underworld, a purgatorio.

Signaling to those above, beyond, a pilgrim's progress;

'From those shades I had a little gone
and was ascending where my master led
when, pointing with his finger, one
cried out; "See, no light is shed
upon the lower of these two;
he behaves like one who is not dead." '

SEVEN

EIGHT BRIEF
CANDLES

I

Attentive to my ill friends, I seek something as obscure as it is crucial. I want to see their lives and deaths, and my own, in a new way. Instead of hanging around waiting for death, with all the accompanying emotional cacophony of those who have merely 'hung around' life—panic, fury, bitterness, depression—I seek a breakthrough; a new freedom, hard won, an emptiness, a giving over. A different beat, a sweeter music, plaintive, even hopeful.

. . .

I know something of that transformation. Not a great deal, but something. It is like a birth, a rebirth. A difficult one, with overtones of barely making it. A breech delivery perhaps? Travail, but then 'rejoicing, for a child has been born into the world.'

. . .

Gloomy skies overhead, clammy weather. One of those days, the nurses say sorrowfully, and shake their heads. I thought to myself, of those days indeed. Let's look for some flowers.

And found them, a clutch of tulips like points of flame—outrageously out of season, barely surviving, like the rest of us, enduring the cold gloomy air. Presented them. 'Oh, what a day!' and then—'Oh, thank you!'

It was a day fit to set New Yorkers running, like raving exiles, toward Peoria or some other unimaginable outpost. Skies shaken in some monstrous joker's hand, muddy, sullen, the world in a bad mood, a chip on the cosmic shoulder—

'Everyone is very ill, no one wants to talk.' Thus went the threnody. On that note I started, through the corridors, up and down the crowded elevators.

First to the emergency ward. There by the youngest, freshest spirit ever to fall under the scythe. He languished there in a cubicle; a musician, alone in New York, his family a world distant in Hawaii. In and out of hospital, released home for a week or two, then the inevitable syndrome staked its claim once more; back he lands, more wan and somber than ever.

He looked at me out of his wide, frightened eyes, lying there in the windowless box reserved for the first third of the triage. A bird of passage, caged.

Let us pray. 'Let us have mercy, first of all on ourselves. Then there might follow mercy toward him.' Otherwise the situation is beyond bearing; looking at him looking at me, a lingering glance that distills, like a tear in the eye of dying Christ, the plight of us mortals.

How dare say to him, or even to myself, 'You are going to die'?

II

But the prize downer of the day was my friend the interior decorator. How say it? Some cosmic joker was at work, bringing down his frame, shaking out his seams.

He too had been released from the hospital, he too was back. Blinded by meningitis, a peculiar and horrid refinement of AIDS, now he was bedridden. And yet, and yet, as I lingered in the room, a nurse entered.

Something happened. No giving up; he was in charge. In unwontedly firm tones, he undertook a rundown of ins and outs, deficiencies and good points of his medical treatment. I was astonished, delighted, to hear this new voice issuing from so wasted a life.

He had not been consulted as to one painful 'procedure.' He shouted, he laid down his demands; that nurses appear as promised, on time, that doctors honor their word. And so on, at some length. Before me, in other words, a new sort of human.

But still, alas, burdened with the old mortality. Nothing new about his dying; as he probably, and I of certainty, knew. During a brief respite at home, the devilish horseman had mounted yet another assault; a new plague spot appeared on the corporeal map, his rectum. There followed all but unbearable agonies and bloodlettings and humiliations consequent to this new onset, as can be imagined. He knew the disease had taken a new turn, and all for the worst. But there was good news too, and it combated the bad; his spirit had taken charge.

III

This man is so close to death, I hesitate in his presence to breathe deeply, for fear of putting his precarious soul to flight.

To speak of beauty is to stretch things more than a bit. He was probably once comely; but for now, he fulfills to the letter the description of the suffering servant in Isaiah; 'No comeliness or beauty did we see in him; a worm and no man. . . . ' AIDS has raked his face to a lazarine corpse; he is covered with purple lesions, his nose blown up like a clown's.

I've seen death in most of its limitless witless guises; but this is extravagant, even for that old skullful of horrors.

He responds not at all to my greeting; not even when I touch his forehead in blessing. I seek information from a nurse; what his condition is, why he shows no response, even by opening his eyes. She reports that he is 'in and out,' and has been so all day. But she accompanies me back to the room, turns on the overhead light, bends over him, says loudly, 'Frank, someone is here to see you.'

He opens one eye wide. The other is half open, out of focus. I offer a blessing, we extinguish the light and depart.

IV

We have among us now and again a drug abuser. One of them is a Jersey construction worker, white, young, fervently tattooed. Weeks ago, Sister warned me: He's going to die hard, of diarrhea, he'll probably never go home.

Sure enough, weeks later, he's still here. At first on his feet, pretty much in charge of time and its vacillations. There was the usual presumption, so hardly given up on; he'd be going home soon.

Now, what a difference! That big frame is attenuated, he's no longer up and about. An old man's tried and untrue look has suddenly descended on him. Time is claiming him, stretching him on its unforgiving rack.

Those eyes turning to me, I knew them well, eyes of the trapped. It was all but settled, there would be no leaving the hospital. But the Himalayan climb toward hope had just begun; he still had far to go, to reach that rare high plateau of pure space, all sky and no ground.

V

A short episode, and by no means unique. The story of a marriage, and a child born.

The marriage breaks up. Years later a revelation: the former husband is gay. Long separated from wife and child, he is ill unto death with AIDS.

The news reached her, the former wife and present mother. (She had taken the burden alone, of raising their son.)

Manifestly, someone must do something; and immediately. She retained her job, an absolute necessity for survival. To it she added another burden, no less exigent. She began nursing the dying man.

After a year of this, she approached me. Would I visit her husband, a former Catholic? I would.

He lived in an old, comfortable, rather shabby brownstone in lower Manhattan. Three rooms, much art work in evidence, a middle class ambience. He was woefully wasted.

We got on well. Talked amicably over tea, a breathable atmosphere. Before I left, he asked me to bless him. And would I return, and bring communion?

A week later, I was back. His wife met me at the door.

I entered the bedroom. In so brief a time, he had failed shockingly; time's short shrift in his face, growing shorter.

With the help of water, he was able finally to swallow the Host. We prayed together, the woman in tears, I nearly so. He seemed comforted. When I said goodbye, he asked me if I would hold his face in my hands.

I took up that nearly empty shell, life on the wane. Strangely enough, dying as he was, I found, and I hope without sentimentality, our predicament strangely alike. Life, the attrition and drought of the years. Simpatico, the soul was intact.

He died within the week.

The burden of these lines is not merely to record, with what feeling I can muster, his passing. I wish first of all to celebrate the wife, her fidelity. The wife who returned to the death bed, despite all (and I am by no means aware of the entire story).

The rupture, and then the unlikely healing. Thus neither anger, aversion, conflict, were allowed the final word.

He received, toward the end, a piece of hallowed bread from my hands. But the communion was a larger and more mysterious reality by far. A widening circle, time and the unknown, he and she and I, the bread of life in the breach of death, the banishing of fear, a healing that surpassed unimaginably the skills of this world.

VI

There he sat, or lay, or wandered about. Still on his feet, his past weighing heavy, by no means a praiseworthy one. Alcohol, drug addiction. And now AIDS. One couldn't miss the message; an Irish hellion once at large, presently and for whatever future, at small.

Small indeed, and bound to go smaller; months ahead, perhaps only a few diminishing weeks, a very knothole to be crawled through.

And he knew it; 'matter of fact' describes him to the hilt.

In hospital, a rosary dangling from a hook on the wall, help of friends who come by, help of daily Eucharist, he's a tamed hellion indeed.

'I know I'm dying.' The tone is level, the look direct. He knew I knew, it was no tidal wave breaking over us. He sat there, his gaze shifted to the window, and beyond. He might be commenting on the most colorless item in the universe; the gray day, gray twilight, nightfall.

'They tell me I'm in the early stages,' dryly. He looks unmarked as yet, none of those telltale lesions, no loss of weight. A vivid carrot complexion, hair in abundance, unmistakable Celtic phiz. And the bluest eyes imaginable, a strange hard-earned innocence. You'd conclude, those eyes on you, ignorant of his dark story—why, mere days before, he'd walked away, sweet six or seven years in the world, hands folded, from a first communion!

AIDS? He looked astoundingly fit, a workman maybe, taking a few days off for a routine checkup.

Yet he knows, the shadow behind the eyes. 'I'm one of the lucky ones, so far.'

Luck of the Irish. Truest luck, a change of heart.

He wants me to know about that profound turnaround. But he's canny, he won't state things directly.

He's a great one for drama. It bursts out of him like wine through a skin. Here he sits or lies flat or paces about, in this strange static temple of harsh lights and right angled corners and mysterious venous potions and half veiled 'facts of life'—facts that, truth told, in his case, amount to an ineluctable outcome, known to all, unnamed except by himself. The courtesy, the reticence, the roundelay; thus the literally unbearable is borne.

He dramatizes his change of heart in ways unexpected and endearing.

'C'mon, I want you to meet someone,' he urges. We start down the hall, he in his kimono and pajamas, by all odds the sturdiest figure in sight.

The meeting in question; an aged wizened bundle of misery. She huddles on a settee in a corner lounge, weeping her heart out. Another woman, also a patient, is doing her best at comforting.

We join the duet. 'Grandma, I want you to meet a friend of mine, a priest.' She perks up momentarily, lifts her head, hanging so pitifully low on her breast, a hundredweight of age.

Moaning, more tears, a flood. 'They won't put me to bed, I'm so tired.'

We hover about, doing our best. He takes her hand. 'They'll be around soon now, Grandma, don't cry.'

The scene is by no means unique; the aged and lorn in any hospital in the land.

Except for this, which lodges the episode in memory. I was led to the scene of an old sorrow, by someone afflicted with a sorrow both new and unforeseen. New, terrible beyond telling; but by no means defeating to the young Irishman. He stood there, companion in woe to a faded November leaf of a woman, forlorn and lost in a land of indefinable sorrow.

He beckoned me along; to help, as he said. What he did not, perhaps could not know, would annotate a Bible.

Among the Irish, the commanding folklore is incised in stone. The priest exists at the beck and call of all comers. But no mortal born, no one, with the arguable exception of God almighty, would presume to help a priest.

How could my friend know the immense help he tendered me?

Someday I'd tell him. Or someone would.

. . .

He went fast. The bald statement is a way of coping; it is also helpless to convey the pain, the downward kick and race of the heart.

The hospital did what it could, then released him. Others needed attention.

His wife, longsuffering amid his ruinous excesses, didn't want him about; for the sake of the children, she said grimly.

Finally, we found him a room in an urban fleabag, a sordid men's shelter near the Hudson River. Best we could do; better at least than the merciless streets.

Within days, the report was grim; he was fading into physical decline and loss of spirit.

I sought him out in a grimy workhouse of a dwelling near West Street, down at the heels, a last stage for the last act of losers, tottering precariously between bottle and needle—and death.

An indifferent warder at the front desk muttered a room number and shuffled off. I mounted the stairs, found the room—and found him not. Nary a trace. No answer to my pounding.

Was he in, was he out? Too discouraged, too far gone, hiding out? I could only slip a note under the door; I've been here, thinking of you, see you again.

He landed back in the hospital, a fare-thee-well.

Now his mind was much afflicted. We sat together for a chat or a smoke, and he no more knew me than daddy Adam. And then he died.

What to make of it? All concerned, as far as could be judged, did their best, given his sorry self, the marriage a wreck, his wife picking up the shards of survival, determined once and for all that the door be shut and the lock in place.

And we did what we could. Hands and skills and the patience that is both hopeful and hopeless, knowing the outcome, holding on. Playing the fictions of time, the sorry crepuscular meantime granted such as he.

And constrained, finally, to let go.

As someone ashore wades out, helps shove off, the vessel light as a leaf riding, the rower finally in command, rising to his stroke, his momentum.

We waved him off finally, in an unimaginable outward tide of mercy.

VII

There was a voluble black man. I met him early on in the game; he was someone new.

He'd gotten AIDS through needles. That was new too, in Greenwich Village, where AIDS was practically synonymous with homosexuals.

Up and down, he was up and down and vice versa, but hardly ever on an even keel. One week he welcomed me like a ghetto brother; the next, he was too weak to remember my name, or too dispirited, or both. And then, the third week, there was other, more ominous news. He was on a survival run, he'd been literally hauled one night, by a kind of medical SWAT team, into the intensive care unit, two floors down.

You have to be there to know what goes on there. Let us understate, and merely say, Intensive Care is no joke, for either side.

Though I've been wheeled into that place of panic and near demise, I will not thereby risk terrorizing the reader. Let the story speak for itself. Our friend, when I sought him out in his new habitat, received me with a kind of desperate warmth, a clutch on a life line. He was bedded in a windowless cubicle; the fourth wall was of glass; it offered the dubious relief of a control panel, winking and blinking away all twenty-four hours, like a sleepless insect eye. Thus his person and condition were immediately visible to the nursing corps. And various instruments were poised, ready to set up a clamor, should his 'vital signs' prove alarming.

His eyes were wild with alarm. He caught sight of me in the doorway, he strained toward me like the last of the living.

'My God, what're they doin' to me?' He raged and fumed and thrashed about. 'Night an' day they keep lights on. They come and go and poke and ast me questions I've answered hours, days ago. I'm so tired, I feel like a side of beef bein' processed. . . . '

Heart failure, I learned, had occurred one night. But someone had been alert and rang the alarm. At that point his heartbeat was so close to zero as to make little difference—except to the conscientious staff, for whom the death of anyone, including a penniless drug addict, was not to be conceded without a fight.

So they fought. And won. But the Queensberry rules! The violations! The sleepless nights, the persistent probings, the needles, the seemingly impersonal comings and goings!

His recovery was under way. This time, at least.

Shaking with anger, he lay there helpless. I listened, nodded like a marionette. Death, one was hard put to remind him, had lost. His fury? It could only be accounted a good sign. He was, for a time, on his way back.

VIII

Yet another Job. Skin and bones, little more. Rendered, reduced. So weak he could summon only a hoarse whisper.

A friend drew me with a nod into the corridor. It appeared that on an earlier, less dreadful occasion, Paul had expressed longing to receive the sacrament of Confirmation, the anointing of adults for the exercise of Christianity in the world.

Paul had never been confirmed. Did he want the usual witnesses to stand with him? No, explained his friend uneasily; Paul was embarrassed at the hiatus in this religious initiation. He would much prefer that no one, not even members of his family, be present.

So it was done, and just in time. Paul was anointed with the holy oil that would make him a staunch member of the faith, on the alert against whatever 'assault of the unholy one.' We prayed together, I read an episode of healing from the gospel. Then we were silent for awhile.

He followed everything with his great sunken eyes, brimming with the pain of letting go. His lips and mouth were bloodied and raw. I thought, by way of a weird contrast, of someone who had eaten a quantity of crushed strawberries.

He sought to stanch the blood with a Kleenex. I received the bloodied paper in bare hands, surely contrary to all the rules, and perhaps to a sensible prudence as well.

But why, I thought, should I dramatize under his alert gaze the dread attached by many to his agony?

It was perhaps a modest version of the kissing of the leper by Francis. More power to me.

I came back a week later; he was comatose. When I came in, calling his name softly, his eyes opened ever so slightly. I held his hands. His lips were caked with dried blood. I heard him murmur, all but inaudibly, 'I'm going home, I'm going home.'

EIGHT

OSCAR—NO STORY WORTH TELLING?

There were a few of whom it could only be said: nothing to say.

Too far gone. They went under like an elevator with cables snapped; down, down, out of sight, a blur, a cry. Death is indeed inventive.

Oscar was like that. If a life could be thought of as a ruinous vertical passage, surely he was dropping fast, at least by the time we met.

One could only stare transfixed, through the small window of the elevator door, as the cube hurtled down, on its way to the great elsewhere.

Everything awful befell him, on the way to Everything.

One week it was his lungs that failed; the next week, his kidneys. There were new, altogether unheard of complications, infections, invasions. In combating which, multiple tubes were inserted in his poor flesh, ingenious apertures devised. One day, I was told, he had contracted something hair-raisingly esoteric; tuberculosis of the liver. That was a new one, even for our liverish world.

He could scarcely speak. Occlusion of the throat. Laboriously and with infinite patience, he was able to swallow a few drops of water; only a few—the sip of a newly hatched bird.

Weeks passed, and no deliverance. What could it mean, that my friend had no story to tell, even to me, who might be thought apt for listening? No story—nothing but this wordless tableau of misery, passing all understanding, all expression.

I had no inclination, after a purgatorial half-hour in that room, to justify the agonies of this interim life, in which poor Oscar wandered like a zombie.

By every law of life, every invocation of the God of life, he should long before have been delivered 'from the body of this death.' What to make of a hanging thread of a man? Who would not stand in awe before this ikon of grief, this scrawl from Job's diary?

He was dumb, very nearly deaf and blind. He lay there, death before death, death refusing death, a cellular resistance which had nothing to do with things vivid or soulful or shouting or hilarious or outrageous, the hues of life and love, the uses of limbs, joy in the seasons, in the wayward gesture of a child—all that evanescent glory we name living—and so naming, take for granted. He was a dumb smoldering log in a hearth lit and warmed for a great celebration.

In the brisk, matter-of-fact way of a hospital, he was taken for granted. Lingering on as he was, not quite dead, he was ... another charge, a responsibility. He must be taken care of; just like any other, including the patient in the next room.

That one, already on his feet, would be going home to his family on the morrow; and must meantime linger, another twelve hours to yawn through.

Thus the nurses made little of what was surely a small thing, the good-natured blather of the recovering man. And then made little of the terrible thing next door, the final rhythm of stupor and groan. Let the trump sound, let the trump pause, they would be there.

Thus help was at hand, and skill, and a certain cool compassion, genuine to the core, but necessarily under strict control.

The help was less visible (mostly to the would-be helper) more problematic, when one entered the room, not as a professional, but a would-be friend.

Then there was little or nothing to say (indeed, there was little to say, by anyone involved, even the most efficient). But still, there might be something to do, some minute innocuous thing. One could draw up a chair and sit on a level with the suffering eyes. And stroke his brow; and do one's best to decipher his poor monosyllables. And not overwhelm the patient with attrition, the words words words of those who, uneasy in such company, stumble about to fill the space, cannot let silence be.

Oscar had no story. Or (roughly the same thing), he was utterly incapable of telling it. No time left, no will or energy; the story dies in the throat.

And yet, I reflect, the Bible does a strange thing from time to time. It guards the story of those denied their story.

With Oscar much in mind, I thought of a parallel. There is another denial of worth and name and dignity in the world—the wipeout of capital punishment. The forced disappearance of a human from this world. It denies in effect that a life is worth telling or hearing, except in execration. Denial that such a one has walked the common ground, breathed the air, known others, comes to anything, anything worth passing on.

Have we understood? Christians worship a God about whom the world declared such things. A God with no story worth telling. A criminal, condemned and legally executed. (That His story was finally told, in no way mitigates the world's contempt.)

This is the 'curse' under which, as Paul writes, Christ fell. He was condemned to death; in the process, his life, example, healing, words, stories—all were stuffed in the grave, as of no possible worth, no claim on attention. *Pereat.* Everything. Let Him be as if he had not been.

Thus was the story of God contemned; the story of the dying One whose words stuck in his throat, toward 'the ninth hour.' How long one must stand there, drawing out the cords of silence, weaving them fine, if he is to comprehend that wordless agony, when the Condemned One, the Man with No Story, hung dying!

. . .

There is more to all this. The judgment of 'no story worth telling' is laid upon lives, from outside, a more or less contemptuous invasion. A system, a culture, is turned to a sword. The weapon is raised. It is at war with civilized (or religious) understanding. It cannot accept that all lives, even the meanest and most criminal, are precious in the sight of God (or the sight of the civilized).

Enough of the judgment of this world, which decides, by sword and fire, noose and shot, war and death row, who shall be denied a hearing.

. . .

This at least can be said, given the terror and nearly unrelieved anguish in that hospital room. No such putrid judgment can be laid against Oscar as degrades the systems of our generation; 'life of no value' (that hideous Nazi judgment on the 'non-productive' of the third Reich.) Nor that other judgment, equivalent when all is said, to the unspeakable first; 'life with no story.'

Sorrow Built a Bridge   167

. . .

I sit with Oscar, I hold his hand, his story hovers on the air. It lingers, even as it lends a glory to his face. It signals true time, which may sound very like a final hour. But in his life, the hour is not final at all; time drags along, draws itself out, like a deadly wire drawn through the guts; a torture, no clean ending.

I listen, I translate as best I can, those groans and would-be words of his. I play human, clumsily, and to little avail. Or so it seems.

And yet his story opens before me, like a volume held by an angel. *Tolle et lege!* No simple or conventional biography. I have access to the hospice reports, they are of little interest. Family, profession, religion even, these are the tags tied to the living; they denote a place in the world, a turf, income, status and the rest. Irrelevant. Something more is at stake; something of essence, mystery.

The Original Story of the one without a story; I think of Isaiah.

> '*He has not stately form or majesty*
> *that we should regard him*
> *nor appearance, that we should be attracted to him.*
> *He was despised and forsaken by all,*
> *a man of sorrows, acquainted with grief.*
> *Like one from whom they cover their face.*
> *He was despised; we found no reason to esteem him.*'

The theme was taken up, later, by others, concerning Another. A like judgment had been laid against this One; nonperson, away away, give us Barabbas.

You must enter the bitterness of that judgment, I tell myself. Then perhaps you will understand how it falls and falls again; a judgment stamped, sealed, delivered, by both powers, church and state. Church, if anything, more adamant, more determined on winning a death penalty before death. I stand with a homosexual, dying of self-contracted disease. The stigma, the verdict; *pereat.*

Harsh matters, harsh, deadly.

A capital judgment indeed. And against the judgment, against its legal pretense, its meticulous moral derangement—our scripture, with altogether direct and chastening irony, has placed its own judgment. It not only vindicates the death (and therefore the life) of the mysterious suffering one spoken of by Isaiah. But it borrows his story, to tell it anew; the story of the death (and therefore the life, and both vindicated) of God in our world.

. . .

I sit beside my friend. If I knew my errand in the world (and indeed, I have only a meager inkling) I could also describe this room; a kind of cave, wherein birth and death are going forward, unimpeded, imaginable. Church and state (alike as two spoiled peas in a pod) have no access here; only midwives and nurses—and the invisible Beloved, to whom the dying one bears a resemblance, uncanny and stark.

NINE

LOST AND FOUND IN THE FLOATING FOREST

After his death, he was slowly to resurrect in my mind, a symbol.

But for now, he lay there in the hospital bed, very much himself; but stricken too.

I began to think of him as emblematic of that procession of the young and doomed, their class, elegance, verve, money, wit, New York edge and polish. All this—and then, the Interruptive Shove.

It was inelegant, a bum's rush.

Something akin to the shove and jolt of subway voyaging, part of the seldom dull journey from here to somewhere. Half the pain is getting there.

But the subway battering is one thing; the chic apartment, the summer lair in the Hamptons or Connecticut, quite another. No swaying, ill-tempered multitudes of the IRT express train tarnish the allure, the ambience; friends, evenings over wine, gently spiteful gossip, classy vacations and weekends. All the perks of the trades. The good life and then some.

. . .

And then, something else, something terrifying. The Interloper. Defying with an utterly inviolable arrogance the conventions, the secure symbols, status, good looks, money, credentials, all the evidence of 'making it.'

. . .

I am meeting him for the first time. And in hospital, a place hardly designed for easeful intercourse of spirit. Friendship does not flourish here; alienation does, and fear and trembling. People enter under duress, hellbent for release, the prompter the better. Who indeed has wit (or witlessness) to praise this sterile overnight caravansary, antiseptic as it is, invasive, allowing no hiding places, the staff often abrupt and grudging?

. . .

He was young, as are all of them, or nearly all. Rangy, over six feet, unconventionally good-looking, alert of eye; the eye of a storm.

There was the matter of the sterile mask, a symbol commonly denounced by the ill. A sign of anonymity; yours, the patient's. Sign of distancing and fear.

One sufferer described the surreal goings on; a flock of marveling medics would shuffle in and surround his bed, masked, for all the world like a Knight of the Klan. They muttered their polysyllabic incantations ('like butchers around hung meat'), they scrawled mysteriously in their pads and departed.

It was bizarre, he said bleakly; one hardly knew; especially if one was in fever, whether he had dreamed the episode or undergone it.

. . .

I put on the mask that first time; it was practically the only time. And then only under duress; because my young friend was flushed with pneumonia, and requested that I don the thing. He dreaded infections from the outside; quite enough invasive crawlers were occupying his person.

There was a touch of the sardonic I found quite comforting. It covered the shock nicely. That he was in shock could hardly be concealed for long; he had been diagnosed that morning. It was AIDS.

I was in a species of shock myself. It was my first venture into the AIDS world. I had dreamed perhaps that the transition could be managed gently, gradually. Hadn't I worked with dying cancer patients for some three years?

I even conjured an image; a child being led step by step, days passing in course, into an adult world. Does death invade that world? Tell the child so, by all means; but ever so gradually, with due regard for the bewilderment, the gradual awakening.

. . .

Then the image dissolves, another forms. There is a face before you, a suffering face and young. Its wearer is being pushed violently out of custom and orbit.

. . .

Another image. A child is assigned, without prelude, in midterm, to a different schoolroom. No friends, no familiar books. The geography of the room is fairly bristling with the unknown. The other students surround one like an impenetrable phalanx, their glances halfway between cruelty and curiosity.

Take the image further. Now the child is transported to another school altogether, in a distant part of town. The world that appears from the bus window—Oh, where am I going?—is totally, terrifyingly unfamiliar. Without landmarks, with an adult hand in his, the child is set down with a thump, on a different planet.

. . .

Death calling the shots. The sterile room, the mask, the gloves, the white robes, the accouterments of a butcher's warehouse, a walk-in freezer, a city morgue. The scene, know it or not, is a revving up for the end. Get ready, take off.

. . .

Donald and I make small talk. Did I know he was an artist? And would I care to see some of his work?

I take up the portfolio. I turn the pages, astonished, delighted; the achievement blazes out.

A running commentary begins. He had returned within the year from Australia and New Zealand. There were honors and perks; a year in residence, a major show in the capital. His work took off, he was earning a tolerable income.

. . .

The work was enchanting. He was of the true artificer tribe, a weaver of reeds and palm and hemp into quasi-human shapes, some on stilt legs, impenetrable, dynastic, ancestral. They were garbed in natural browns, grays, muted rusts. Their limbs curved gently or were twisted in menace, they loomed from a giant height, protective or fierce, angelic or demonic.

There were large photos of his museum show in Melbourne. I saw a long gallery, some sixty by twenty feet, shapes recumbent and standing, a mysterious procession, masks, majesties. An assembly of demigods, recognizably (but barely) human. An exodus of sorts; or perhaps an entrance rite.

He called the assembly 'Floating Forest.' In the midst was suspended a hammock or portable cot. On it rested a figure wrapped in silence, like an ear of corn in its husks. It was regal and timeless, hieratic, an imperial mummy attended by the living. Before and after, attending the mysterious corpse, other figures stood or walked, their appearance both protective and threatening.

Was the artist miming the fate of all, or his own?

I ventured, 'The dead figure walks again, in spite of all. You seem to have come on a resurrection theme.'

Then, 'I wonder if your intuition went ahead of events, and you knew in some way, years ago, what was coming.'

He said nothing. It was, after all, only three hours after the diagnosis had fallen.

In a piece he wrote two years later, shortly before his death, I came on this:

> 'What was gnawing at the most basic level of my physical being began to express itself in 'Floating Forest.' Three large figures constructed of handmade cast papers emerged. I was surprised at myself, feeling I had bitten off more than I could chew. . . .
>
> One piece was a sleeping figure covered with paperback I'd collected in Arubem Land. It was resting in a dream canoe and was very peaceful and gentle.
>
> Next came a nightmare tableau comprised of three elements; a flying sled impaled with sharpened sticks, a bound figure

covered with bottle-brush pods and pierced with twigs. And finally a huge menacing cockroach that hung over the other two. . . .

The last piece was 'Survival,' a hollow, winged creature with its innards totally exposed. Layers of fiber unwound from its head as it flew—illusions lost in flight.

The environment was exhibited in Adelaide, Melbourne and Sydney. It was very well received and thousands wandered through it. I couldn't believe I'd done it.

For me the meaning became very clear two years later, in October of 1982, when I was diagnosed as having AIDS. . . .'

. . .

I departed for Latin America for four months. Donald had rough going during my absence. In and out, out and in the hospital. Between bouts he functioned at home, but only with help.

One day there was a call from him; welcome home, and would I stop by?

The change in him was like a shutter coming down on the day. He dragged himself to the door and greeted me with a smile like a cheerful skeleton's. Thinned down now, thin as a walking bone. And those telltale splotches on the face, deep brown on pallor; the mold of death.

We talked and talked, making the best of things; he offered and was able to steep, a cup of tea. The effort was incongruously huge.

'I sleep until near noon, and it's three in the afternoon, and I'm exhausted,' he said.

I asked about his work. Some half-done things; he dismissed them with a shrug. 'But one thing's to the good. My doctor's favorite sport is dunning me for money. I've offered him a few things in lieu of cash; and he's agreed. So that's an ape off my back.'

It was one thing to be dying, I thought. But to be plagued for payment, in return for services that, truth told, alleviate little or nothing?

It was all loony.

. . .

He was to last awhile longer, that was all. No guarantee of 'prosperity and long life,' as the Bible describes the sojourn of the patriarchs. Age thirty-five; his biography entitled: Decline and Fall.

. . .

So Donald wove beforehand, like the necromancer he was, the drama of death and life. I picture him, long after his death, a browned, loincloth-clad solitary, seated in lotus position in the door of a cave. He is weaving his rushes and grasses, weeds and flowers, into wondrous forms, a tapestry that rustles with dry speech even as he weaves.

The work turns and turns about in his hands. Figures emerge. And words, words float above the figures like a talisman in a wind.

What do they say? He knows, but he cannot or will not say.

And if he could, or if he would, his words would pass us by, incomprehensible as the dry rustling of the weeds and leaves in his hands.

His figures speak a language native to him, native to the dead, a language not of this world.

. . .

His art abides; it stands by him. In its integrity, its mystery, his art rendered his terrible illness at least relatively bearable.

Whereas, if his illness were taken alone, borne alone, without that penumbra of mystery and meaning, catastrophe might well have pitched him into a Gehenna of despair. Where many, not so favored or enlightened, have landed.

Maybe, I surmise, something like this, a convergence of insights, symbols, hunches verified—something like this might describe a way of coping with disaster; events touching all, not just the AIDS-stricken.

. . .

After a month's absence, I phone him. He is very weak, has had yet another terrible episode in hospital. Will I come over, he longs to read me a few jottings he has been setting down.

It sounds like the first notes of a swan song.

. . .

This occurs to me. Those stricken are under a mysterious summons. They are 'going on ahead.' Something like our artist, who wove his rushes, more or less unconsciously, by a law blind to his eyes and clear only to his fingers; wove his own future—for encouragement and warning and dire sign.

A few years later, the artist would face death. But something else happened, as he came to realize, slowly and with terror and much trembling of spirit.

．．．

I was gone from New York five months. To put matters shortly, statistics instead of tears, every AIDS patient I had visited in St. Vincent's had died in the meantime, except my friend the artist. The bell tolled for every one, with his sole exception.

Perhaps he had a stronger will to survive, perhaps dietary care helped. In any case, he wasn't winning, he was bartering time.

．．．

I was like a stunned calf, hearing the news; name after name, all gone. It was as though all normal sense of time had flown the coop. Time and its sane clocks had gone mad. What time was it, in the real world? Had I been away fifty years or five months? Everyone had died.

In Argentina I had read again *A Hundred Years of Solitude*, that straight-faced mockery of time and reason.

For me, the book came weirdly true in my hands. A cosmic clock had indeed gone cuckoo.

I moved in dream. The people I knew and loved were going about the business of living, sedate, sensate, on their feet. But they moved in the wavering slow motion of underwater trolls walking in sleep. You could not talk, you could only gesture feebly, witlessly, reading lips like the lips of fish.

And every gesture was of farewell.

This is something of how I felt, on my return to New York. Only one left, of all who had been ill, in and out of hospital.

．．．

In those early ventures of mine along the AIDS ill, almost every move was in the nature of a first clumsy try. Would one be welcomed, would one be shown the door? How would a greeting, even an innocuous statement, be taken? It was all quite chancy. So much had to be taken on faith, on both sides.

. . .

They land in the hospital; it's like the aftermath of a riptide. The sailing was sweet at first, a cruise in the gentlest of seas. Then came the storm and shipwreck.

Pardon the inextricable metaphors, it's like a tangled net cast ashore after a storm. Like the knotted nets I come on, along the beaches of Block Island. Salted and sandy and cold; the sea waters, like two hands of Triton, knot the cords about and around. Combustive complication, I fret to myself.

. . .

First to the complication. Most of the ill at St. Vincent's are Catholics. The connection holds, in an increasingly vague way, between the faith of patients and the institution.

Gay and Catholic. Irreconcilables. No news to anyone; the official church atmosphere in New York, as it touches on 'their kind,' is a very whiff of brimstone.

So the following is predictable when I venture into a hospital room. Alarm flags are hoisted—by patient, family, lover. Panic, anger, war. In sum, and at very least, who needs you?

Another complication; the matter of family. A considerable matter indeed, when the chips are down. And, as is probably common knowledge, Catholic families, at least as far as elders are concerned, are not great or notable homophiles.

A subject like gayness, frowned on by the ecclesiastical mighty, is not likely to sponsor huzzahs in the front parlors of Queensborough. Not likely. Especially when the church, again and again, traces a blessing (powerful big medicine, this) on the ingrained phobias of Irish or Italian or Polish or German (or anything) Catholics.

. . .

They gather about the bedsides of their stricken ones; parents, sons, brothers and sisters, lovers, wives. Sorrow, disorientation, anger, fear, dread of the unknown. The lovers have it hardest of all, making their unsteady way through the gantlet of church, state, family, neighborhood, job, housing, life in sum. Including, as word gets about and their cover is blown, the feral looks laid on them in the corner deli.

And then, as if this weren't enough, in comes this priest—about whom, if one has ear to the ground, one has heard a few things. So what good can come of this?

. . .

As to the good, or what remote part I might have in its making, I wouldn't sweat a bet on an inflated nickel.

Who could waste thought on an abstract good, disguised ego at best, manipulation at worst? The only good I could understand lay there, suffering flesh and bone, a life ill unto death, the human interrupted, normalcy and expectation gone awry.

. . .

AIDS; the mysterious immunity system of humans breaks down.

Do we have a useful symbol here?

Indeed there are enough learned tomes at our disposal to blot out the sun. They tell us in one way or another that the immunity system of an entire civilization is collapsing.

. . .

Imagine a people so enchanted with death, that masked charlatan who boasts a curative for any and all ills—so won over by his wheedling and dealing as to summon his services on behalf of all the living! Including ourselves. Come unholy spirit of nukes and nightmares!

In such a hypothesis, of course, the Son of God who showed quite another way, who from being eternally immune rendered himself vulnerable to death—is necessarily declared passe. There are newer, more rational and persuasive, less inflictive and demanding gods at beck and call.

. . .

The gods of death. Their tactic is the breaking down of the promise of immunity from death, the destruction of hope; the hope of that immunity which bears as many names as newborn children across the world; Faith, or Grace, or (a title worthy of a princess) Love of God and One Another.

Let no one be immune! is the cry of non-hope. Let hearts be hardened! Let compassion be obliterated! Let all be persuaded, by hook and crook, by bomb and brutality, that death is in effect a good way of life!

. . .

Goodbye, dear friend, artist, lover of life. You taught me, by no rote or ferule, the hardest art of all, the least esteemed in a time of chagrin and distemper, the hardest art of all—the art of dying well.

In a sense, the art could not be taught, at least by the common methods open to practitioners of medicine or religion. You taught by welcoming me to your agony (even as I welcomed you to my home and table). Most of all, best of all, you taught by example. So you stand in my mind; those Erebus eyes of yours looking the darkness in the face, that deadpan equanimity that dares the malignant powers to do their damnedest, and so puts them to rout.

TEN

IKON OR IDOL:
AND ONE
WHO CHOSE

Y ou got the idea quickly, or you did not. The idea: it was no one's business but his own, this dying.

Which in a sense included you too; your dying in due time was like his, your own. A subtle parallel there, not of his devising, though his eyes verified it beyond reasonable doubt.

In any case, he welcomed me at the door, moving slowly as though objects might unaccountably be in the way, a kind of eggshell effect. The thin, graceful frame, the face patrician, charming, even after the ravages of the months.

Tragedies could be referred to with calm, one sensed, not because the worst was over (it was not)—the worst was simply present, here and now, a stone in the guts, something referred to as life. One teetered about on the edge; spongy ground underfoot, worse to come. As to coping, what better idea was there?

There was the business of the church. Born Episcopal, become Catholic in his youth. Then recently, 'due to events and pronouncements,' this dryly, 'returned to the old fold.' Now Episcopal again, and after years and years, not only as a Catholic, but working for the hierarchy!

It struck him as funny. It struck me as something other than.

But to get off that; which commonly gets nowhere, as both he and I knew. On this issue, which for him was an issue of faith, then of being abandoned, there was simply nothing to be done, and less to be said. One endured. There was a history of such endurance, and it eventually won out; which is to say, it survived, and along with it, whatever might be accounted human and decent in the church as well. That church and such as we would meet again. When a great many condemnations and pronunciamentos and a vast measure of hypocrisy had had its day; and with the day, had withdrawn.

There were hints and starts of a deep personal faith. No great deal made of it. He said calmly at one point, 'A year ago I tried to take my life.'

It was the dead calm of a death row. One had endured everything on the list of life's outrages; what worse could there be in store?

Spoke of prayer. 'Sometimes I ask God to lay off, enough being enough. At other times, I shrug in his direction, do your damnedest.'

We sat there in the living rooms, making the small talk that makes a death sentence bearable, for awhile. The setting was genteel, well accoutered, the scent of old money, old culture, understatement.

I proposed he should signal me when the end of the visit was desirable; I didn't want to exhaust him. 'Nothing of the sort, I love visitors.' He lit a smile that would break the heart of an executioner.

· · ·

This is a pause, for honor's sake. It is by no means in the common run of experience, that someone who is manifestly dying, and knows it to the hilt, all the bitterness, the lost chances, the years not to be—and has, moreover, within a matter of months, lost one most loved—it is not common, let us say, that such an outcome of a life most promising is accepted with heartbreaking grace. Taken as a matter of course, a matter of courtesy. Matter of delight, that a stranger should appear at his door, and wish him good fortune (or at least less ill fortune). And be so received that the visitor accounts himself not only welcomed, but blessed.

There were photos of his dead friend on a nearby table; he referred to them with no great emotion. Their subject, beloved as he was, was gone, that was all. The photos were not the friend, they were the poorest of substitutes. Still, given everything, better than nothing. This was the tone, nuanced, dry.

It brought to mind the deaths Yeats wrote of, in the Irish great houses; no whining, death in patrician style. Noblesse oblige; you went as you had lived.

The image was softened by time and the access of another style. It was as though old statuary of Ireland, horses and their riders, had been softened and made permeable by time. The outlines are blurred in many weathers and seasons, the figures humbled. Stiff backs bend a bit. Can one be in charge forever, even through surrogates, descendants? The great ones too must die, a lesson long in the learning.

Well. We are sitting in the living room of a New York apartment, year 1987. He had been an undoubtedly elegant figure in something known as the 'communications world.' Upper middle class, a pro. Settling in, a lover, an apartment, the New York kudos that, a certain status attained, come one's way.

There's something of a . . . creeping Protestantism gets into one's thinking at such times. Meeting his like. Knowing the church, 'as presently constituted,' simply isn't working, for him, for conscience and instinct and the heart's ebb and high tide.

One thinks of oneself, not in a defunct or debased psychological way. But in the way of the Christian ikons, or the Buddhist, any of these. Which is to say (it sounds electric as a shout in a closed tomb)—something of one's own native dignity, evoked from the lives and works of saints. Those one will never, up close, emulate; but will, come what may, admire. And therefore and thereby take hope.

'Admiration.' I think it a good start. The turning of the mind's eye, circling, and focusing, and ... appreciating. Standing there, in a kind of wonderment. The conclusion, which brings such joy: I can do something like this; nothing of the same moment (which is not the point, except as ... admiration). But something like.

And that 'something like' is accepted, welcomed. Not that I am to be great, or celebrated or famous (those fatuous sops of the kultcher). But at all costs I will walk in my own skin, and hearken to my voices.

I reserve that to myself. Because—I admire someone, some few, who have so walked. Impinged on my imagination is a certain image of the human, long lasting, verified in blood and sweat (and a Buddha smile)—'grace,' as they say, 'under pressure.'

It all becomes easy, or at least less damnably difficult. Due to the admiration. The one(s) admired, who are one's true ancestry, and perhaps, though one cannot know, one's progeny.

There has to be another appeal than the one which once worked, or works perhaps here and now, for some. But not for oneself, not by a long shot. Put it thusly: the church no longer functions as a court of appeals against the monstrous world. It has joined forces with the world, it collaborates, in a sense we have learned something of. It is the ally of the prosecutor, it is one with the hanging judge, it poisons the ears of the 'jury of peers.'

Difficult. Beyond words. The rhetoric, the history of the rhetoric, is incised in stone, and the stones are a veritable Stonehenge, they have stood for so long, they exert that pressure and persuasion of survival: 'We are the court of last appeal, there is no other.'

How many Joans of Arc?

They said in tones that plainly threatened death by the torch; You are wrongly, willfully persuaded, misled.

And she could only cry out, 'God is my witness. God and my voices. I must obey them.'

We are not of her mettle. But it would seem as though we are being led, much against our will, in a like direction.

On the one hand, there is quite literally no one to 'admire'; the ikons are inferior, their painters have not preceded their work with prayer and fasting. We are being ill-instructed by— I leave it to you.

For all that, granted all that, there is a God. There are, here and there and everywhere, and at all times past, holy ones. I can choose among them, or be chosen, it comes to the same thing. And be still in their presence, allowing the aura, the aureole, that standing waterfall of humanity we name holiness, to inundate my soul.

I would be like that, him or her; and so become myself.

It seems to me this is godly activity, favored by God. I cannot but obey my voices.

The ikon versus the idol; a fruitful contrast. In reality, in understanding. The church as ikon, the church as idol.

The first is life giving. The blessing and beckoning hand. The admiration which is true worship; 'I would be like you, you have drawn me.'

The second as reproof, condemnation, death dealing. The Church acting as judge; and then the inevitable outcome, which is never or hardly ever acquittal.

We must break the idols. Scripture says it. So do the Buddhists. (If you meet the Buddha on the way, kill him.)

'I left the Catholic church.' Nothing to admire. Ikons? Idols.

The sweetest revenge against the idols is to go on, calmly venerating the ikons.

Sweet; as long as it is understood that those who presume to take revenge, will have revenge exacted of them.

The vengeance of the idols? No one in Robert's quaking shoes needs instruction on this. Vengeance is mine, say the idols.

. . .

Let us not yield to gnosticism. The idols and the ikons are not equal entities. Any more than Satan and the Lord are equal adversaries.

The clue of the inequality, which is of substantial moment, lies in the conquest of death, versus the dealing of death. In this regard, my friend clearly prevails.

The contest was never to be understood as between him and the idols. Robert was merely the surrogate of the Presence. It is this humiliated understanding which makes of him so winsome and modest a stand-in. He knows, in a sense that utterly surpasses psychology, who he is. And who he is not.

This also makes it a joy to be in his presence. Even while one is sensing, too, the sting of death, in one's own flesh. Friendship with the dying is never (if so needs saying) an easy drift downstream.

Well, he invites me to lunch in a week. We shall see what we see.

. . .

We ate at one of those Greek coffee houses in Chelsea; they seem, he said, 'to be stamped out all over the city.' And then;

'someone said there's a cooking school in Athens that has ten specialties. Now they're all over the world.' And I, 'You'd say maybe, that the Ph.D. grads come to Chelsea, the flunks to the Upper West Side?'

Time went on, I was so moved by his gentle self-possession, I took courage to probe a bit. What were his thoughts on friendship, its cost, its endurance; and most painful of all, its loss? The subject, I surmised, was of as great moment to him as to me.

Much talk ensued. He confessed he'd lost several friends due to his illness.

The admission struck a kindred note; so had I lost this or that blessed friend, due to certain meddlesome tendencies I had cultivated over the years. A strange confluence of crises, a strange likeness in outcome.

I was led to suggest that losses by no means composed the whole story. Other, unpredictable outcomes graced one's life. Strangers became friends, walked toward one, offered support, declared one's actions of crucial import to themselves. And a number of old friends came even closer.

He agreed. The worst time of all, he said somberly, befell him in the course of his lover's dying. 'We were both ill that year; I was a bit stronger and cared for him. Then he was taken to the hospital. And the friends who'd never once in the course of our illness entered our home, suddenly appeared in the hospital. How explain it? It was as though they were looking for a kind of safe house. And the apartment, for some reason or other, was unsafe.'

In my account, the crisis rose from a different event, but took a strangely similar turn. A number of friends simply couldn't stomach civil disobedience; 'This time he's gone too far.' Then came that species of absence that makes the heart grow somber. They never so much as bade me farewell. Neither rhyme nor reason was offered. They simply vanished.

on our medical treatments. It's clear to me that because he has so little money, he's getting second- or third-rate attention.'

And a bit later, another episode in the same vein; the so to speak better within the bitter. 'My roommate is an actor; jobs these days of course are spotty. Two weeks ago, mysterious symptoms started. He panicked for awhile, something was obviously wrong, he might soon be needing all sorts of medical help. He'd better hire out for a 9 to 5 job.

'Sure enough, a week later he was diagnosed; AIDS, that old bugger. But he now has medical benefits, just under the wire, so to speak.'

Still later: 'I count eighteen friends who've died in three years.'

All in all, a most unassuming and matter-of-fact Job.

. . .

He beckoned me into the kitchen one day; a series of prizes, wall plaques and such, were on display. Inscriptions testified to the esteem of colleagues for his radio and TV productions.

'Ecce,' with a grandiose gesture, 'the encomia of a well spent life. Alas, alack, if that were all!

'It wasn't. Certain types, my type, were shown the door some time ago. A blind bat could get the message; Get lost, you guys, posthaste.

'Well, I'd had it. I packed up these goodies and sent them back to their donors. And you know what? Not a word, not even an angry word. They shipped them back again. I can scarcely bear to look at them; maybe the next repository is the trash bin.'

And again one day, without prelude, 'I suppose such misbegotten types as I will be hated until the last day.' Words to that effect. And as to their deadly accuracy, I could have little doubt.

· · ·

It was like that game we played as children. You tossed dice to a board, your pilgrim moved backward or forward in accord with the cast.

One step forward, three or four back, his game too. There followed a scouring series of setbacks in his quest for survival. He announced that he was consulting a lawyer with a view to 'winding up my affairs.' I had not previously heard, among the very ill, things put in so dry a fashion. It set up an echo in my mind; he might have been a revenant Stringfellow, the astringent Episcopal tone was so alike.

· · ·

A few weeks later, talk turned for the first time to his funeral arrangements. He approached the 'dies irae' topic without preliminary, the usual half-smile in place.

Would I be inclined to take part in the celebration? 'I know in view of local regulations, many Roman priests would be reluctant...' His voice trailed off, courtesy allowed the conclusion to be my own.

I averred, 'But this one isn't!'

He seemed reassured and dropped the subject. Perhaps he'd only been testing me. 'Well, in any case, I told the rector to keep things cool, no long-winded homilies, five minutes or so. It's nice to know you'll be there on the altar; please play it as you want.'

. . .

The old ache of devastation comes over me, yet once more.

Now he could barely pick up the phone; and when he did, the voice was like a whisper from another world. 'It's terrible, these crashing headaches. The other morning I woke up, my head was like a split melon.

'I started a morning prayer, what a prayer. I was screaming at God like a maniac, Why? Why? The neighbors must have thought I was going stark mad.'

The foregoing, be it known, from a commonly self-contained gent, once very much in command of life, its visitations and permutations. No longer. A terrible beauty is born.

. . .

And I—what can I summon against the night? It claims the autumn sky like the slowly stretching wing of a carrion bird. All I can summon—these poor words set down, my thoughts, memories, travail.

These and a conviction: that he is moving toward a greater mercy than this world can offer.

That the final act in the drama is not wrought by that loony body snatcher, bunched up on a wintry bough.

. . .

He was conveyed to hospital shortly thereafter, much against his will. What else to do? He resisted to the end what is currently known, in a sulfurous phrase, as 'aggressive intervention.'

And died within the week.

It was yet another blow. I went reeling about for some hours, picking up, here and there, pieces of life; for all the world like someone deprived of all good sense.

ELEVEN

THE DREAM, THE DREAMER

I

First as to the Dream, and its failure.

It is no news (and yet it is most tragic news), many of those afflicted with AIDS are falling out of the Dream, even as they take the tumble into death.

The Dream is of immortality, of youth as immortal. And for many, a dream of youth claims a setting of achievement, money, life in a precious setting; the ego and its pavane.

Certain among us must (the imperative is urgent) be ensconced in a befitting decor; clothing, dwelling, food and drink, all of the highest quality. Starved faces may appear wraith-like at the window, hands may beat at the door. Cries too are heard, third-world cries, competing myths and slogans, persistent and loud as to political and ethical and economic inequities.

The voices and their owners are furious at the spectacle of these 'haves.' They attach harsh names to our Dream and its Dreamers; selfish, un-Christian, inhuman, parasitic.

To speak of gays, the reaction of the third world tends in many respects to run with the hostile domestic current. Third world or first; Down With Them! The envy, hatred, excoriation, religious ousting, biblical denunciations mount, an all but universal chorus.

. . .

Perhaps we have a clue here to the mauling of gays by many 'revolutionary' governments. Their leaders, vociferously condemning nearly every aspect of capitalistic life, strangely echo the hatreds of North America and Europe—gays, the pampered darlings of economic arrangements shot through with injustice. In consequence, no room for such, in a 'virile,' young, self-created, revolutionary society.

The point, I take it (as thoughtful gays take it), is surely a serious one.

And it is just at this point of revolutionary exclusion, when old hatreds don new fatigues, that the church is called to intervene, to register its discernment, translation, objection. Raising for instance a question: what revolution can claim credence, when it drags along in its wake ancient hatreds, under whatever plausibility?

Alas, the church does no such thing. It echoes in fact the prevalent sentiment and frenzies of the world; whether first, second, or third. The gays are seized upon as a kind of universal political solvent. Solve finally their presence, their very existence.

Shall we call them Gypsies, Jews?

. . .

I thought of meeting points, where understanding might blaze anew. Nuclear weapons, we are informed by implication, 'protect' gays as well as all others; this is perhaps the most wearying and redundant political statement of recent history. Under the umbrella of terror, all make do, cowering blissfully.

A truer evaluation, one which very few arrive at (especially in light of a fairly comfortable existence) would persuade that nukes enslave us all.

. . .

Indeed the content of the Dream, all said, is decreed by... nukes. The images shift with disconcerting speed, from visions of sweetness and light to febrile nightmare; from material comfort to terror. Consumer goods induce soul numbing, a 'Star Wars' scenario opens for an indefinite run in a culture of the absurd.

According to its confabulators, the scenario (dolce vita, terror) will pump out the determining images for centuries to come. The Dream will verify the dominance of technique, of appetite and quick satiation, of freedom honored in theory (and progressively scorned in practice). The future will be the present, immensely hyped up, concentrated.

Thus the images that claim us will rule our children also. (Presuming the blessing of progeny. The scenario presupposes this, and simultaneously endangers it. Like the monster in Inferno, the prospect both begets and eats its offspring.)

. . .

Thus a self-contradicting Dream makes slaves of us, keeps us inert and victimized, holds our children and ourselves hostage.

And yet we are instructed by the highly placed Smilers to keep smiling away; as though the dollars in our pockets or the brains in our heads were still workable, negotiable, a sound tender. As though in plain fact our world were not raving mad in its chief parts. And driving us mad, as the admission price to the Fun House.

. . .

Another, related matter occurs. In a peculiar and spurious visitation, the Dream subsumes certain images from the past and presents them as valid here and now. Images of nationalism, just wars, liberating wars, myths of sacred nationalism, religious-civic fealty. It focuses on these with reverential attention, awakens myths and hopes, achievements, possibilities, visions of normalcy—all of which at one time held a certain restricted validity, all of which are simply gone with the wind; the wind over Hiroshima.

. . .

Fixation and distraction, together.

The Dream denies and suppresses certain truthful, even crucial aspects of life and its tasks; aspects of danger, resources of moral courage, the necessity of risk-taking, occasions when the human simply must step forward and give and give—even its blood. Or be shamed.

Perhaps most destructive of all, the Dream lulls, diminishes, devalues a history of moral courage. The story of citizens who, in our American past, crossed lines, spoke up, trespassed forbidden ground—and so saved the day.

The loss of such history must be accounted an incalculable disaster. It unmoors, leaves us adrift in a culture that peddles a bizarre blessing on amnesia, selfishness, appetite. Losing our history, we lose our minds.

II

In its classical American version, the Dream conjures up a famous trinity of ikons; a pie baked by a mom. About her there floats, like a Shekinah, an American flag.

. . .

The story concerns another version of the Dream. . . .
A story of a friend, a valued and long-term one.
Shortly, between young friend, half Galahad, half wimp, and myself (half and half also) a peculiar split came down. The friendship fell in two.
It appeared at the same time that in other respects Jeremy's fortunes improved notably. He was growing rich. Condos, investments, travel to Europe and elsewhere; wherever the dollar was sound and the sun at high noon.
Item: a New York town house, title clear.
Item: market bullish. And finally
Item: impeccable health, good looks, such charm as would transform Nemesis and her lightnings into a veritable lady Liberty, smiling her big harboring smile.

. . .

Jeremy's dream, it developed, did not supplant the American one. Indeed no. Mom was there; the pie, succulent, awaited.

But as to Mom, vanished was the apron, the faintly harassed look of maternal servitude. In time, she was transfigured; a twelve-armed Shiva. And her Pie grew into a very cornucopia of creation.

. . .

Indeed, all, all was changed. There fell on the Dreamer and his new entourage of friends a kind of mystical blur. They were rendered all but immortal.

Death? That horrid rumor? It was no more than a fetid whiff on a perfumed breeze.

. . .

A new spirituality prevailed, I was informed. If the ineffable could be subject to the vulgarity of mere gags—this wonder was known as 'Christian Capitalism.'

Due regard was thus paid to the niceties of grammar, which attach to adjectives (even to those graced with a capital letter), a merely modifying force. In casu: adjective 'Christian'; 'Capitalism' noun.

And on that noun, as on a very Rock of Ages, our friend placed every available secure and sound American Christian buck.

. . .

Of the fabulous derring-do of Americans in the great aula where dreams are dreamed, there is no need to linger. Dreams by night, deeds by day—the motto is an imperative, it subsumes the Decalogue.

But form first, as Aquinas would say. The motto is first and foremost a message to the mind. Conduct follows; the addiction to pragmatic bloody rough-and-tumble, from wars to Wall Street.

. . .

Jeremy dreamed and dreamed. In the manner of a jealous lover he claimed the Dream for his own. But the Dream was too jealous, and returned night after night—to claim him. It came in many guises; as Shekinah, covenant, coven of spirits. In time it grew exigent, insatiable, addling. Had day become night, or vice versa? The Dream swamped time and attention and imaginative powers.

. . .

The Dream also brooked no rivals. It evicted aspects of his life once judged central.

Chief among these was the matter of religious faith. He had been a believer; in his young days, a fervent one. But the dreams shook its hoary locks; no. It had in hand other rewards, other symbols; it shortly imposed a contrary ethic.

One world fell apart; but he was comforted, for another simultaneously took form.

. . .

The speed and thoroughness of the transformation were astonishing. What had been a kind of Gibraltar, a founded rock of tradition, conviction, discipline—these dissolved to a mere nostalgic phase, a puff of memory. A history both long and varied, a procession of saints and scoundrels, wise and foolish, laggards and equipoised (but wearing a like look, speaking a common tongue)—they passed him by; better, he waved them away.

And along with such visitants and all they stood for and stood by, went the obscure beckoning known as faith.

. . .

A new world took shape. It included its own coterie and chorus, and a new philosophy. There was the matter previously alluded to, of 'Christian Capitalism.' There were instructors, much talk of 'relevance' and 'renewal.' His mind was shortly cleansed of the impeding past.

. . .

Once, before the Dream prevailed, I accounted myself a close friend. Then the change befell; those of my ilk shortly were rendered insubstantial, obstructive even. And he, a cool-eyed, twice-born neo-realist (the Dream is bullish on 'reality'), now offered to friendship and its dead graces only the frigid comfort of decent burial.

. . .

The Dream, like every True Faith, is self-defining, self-enclosed, self-justifying. This is its strength. Only the chosen initiate is capable of sounding its inner depth, its riches and rewards, its absolutely irrefutable standing.

The rest of us, pushed outside, judge the Dream only at distance; and hardly dispassionately. We think to understand, and we can only mourn, for our understanding is made liverish by memory.

We see only a contagious and frivolous strut known as 'improved life style.'

. . .

To Jeremy we existed only as images of the newly dead, vivid and somewhat painful, but fading. Quick, quick the fading. New realities crowded in, the shadows fled. He faced a rising sun and its shower of gold.

. . .

Even the image of death did not encompass our humiliation. We were worse than dead. In this new dispensation, such as we were accounted ... simpletons. We had missed the boat; the galleon of the Dream, its prow ascending straight up, ready to seize the riches of the sun.

. . .

Another image.

Outside our ken, exempt from recriminative regrets, stood intact and full-blown a form of American quackery; the formula whereby piss-wet straw is transformed, with a snap of finger and a magician's mutter, into gold.

. . .

We could be indignant at this—and be damned. We could account ourselves betrayed, and fret as we pleased. The facts did not favor us, if we were so foolish as to push our case.

The facts had been snatched from our hands; they belonged to the landscape of the Dream, a closed garden. From which, it goes without saying, commoners were accounted trespassers, and liable as such.

We might choose to take a perverse pride in our loneliness, our loss. We could square our shoulders, mutter something about 'bigger than all that,' 'success being of no moment,' a 'higher calling,' and so on. Dim consolation.

. . .

We were stuck. And he had luckily become unstuck. Here, properly understood, was ample matter for discomfiture on our part; and on his, of ego stroking.

. . .

We were indeed stuck; the long and short of it. A matter of Christ dwelling in the same world as ourselves, Christ and his demands, his remindings, his naggings at the edge of the mind; a sorry business at best.

The inhibitions implied, the limits, the downright inefficiency, the confounding and reproof, the blessed are you and woe to you, the dovetailing of means and ends—these were our burden.

Jeremy, it appeared, knew no burdens. He knew only freedom and fun.

. . .

I tread carefully here. Beyond doubt, the abovementioned Christ, His way in the world, forbade us access to the Dream.

And yet it must be confessed, only by fits and starts could we be called meek, obedient, single of mind.

We were more like ragged, wide-eyed beholders of the shower of gold. The Dream was off limits, fenced off. But there we stood, some of us more than a little envious; the shower had not fallen on us.

. . .

Time plucked him from our side. We could brood over offenses suffered or imagined, judge with harshness our former friend. But these are sorry occupations for humans; and we knew it.

Our judgments, darkened as they were by chances lost (by envy?), fell on Jeremy. But in rare moments we knew a like lust was lodged in us too; we loved what we purported to despise. Dolce vita.

. . .

We resembled, more closely than was easily admitted, those in the gospel who looked back, having put hand to their vocation. They heard, at right hand and left, other voices, good fortune, lovely event.

The plowboys were not comforted. They sighed and trudged on, haltingly, with half a heart.

The Dream whirled about them like the demons of Saint Anthony.

. . .

Let us confess our picayune vision, our obsession with observance and undiscipline, our half-heartedness along the way chosen. (But never truly chosen, once for all.) We too are Americans; the Dream dazzles us like a whore's dance.

Alas, we know that the way we chose (or were chosen for), that 'way' of the early Christians, offers few consolations and even fewer rewards. Sometimes, little more than companionship in misery.

A further confession. We are uncertain of the road, less certain than need be. Few of us read the map well, few can claim access to the One who said, 'I am the way.' Few in consequence point the way with conviction and walk it with single mind.

. . .

What meantime of the Dreamer? His story worsens. In ways that are unpredictable (and yet have become utterly predictable), the Dream turns to a nightmare.

To such a Dream that is, even to a paradisiacal one, there comes an awakening. And to the wakening their attaches invariably a modifier: 'rude.'

* * *

On a certain day, fortune, inexplicably out of all control, pitched the Dreamer bodily out of the lofty urban bower in which his Dream had incubated.

We deal in images, a limiting method. Yet the images exempt us from dreary forensic detail. Our friend, to put matters shortly, landed hard.

The diagnosis was delayed for some months. Meantime, his state was vaguely disturbing. He was neither fully awake nor solidly out of things, neither bounding with health nor seriously ill. Distempered certainly, strangely out of sorts, lacking joy in the superabundant emoluments of the Dream.

* * *

Was he a young Hamlet perhaps, both magnetized and repelled by choices?

No, after considerable thought, not that.

No Hamlet. America and its Dream are inhospitable to knuckle-gnawers, to weighers of moral jot and tittle. We are not a nation of doubters; our genius runs to surefooted doers, impatient at the starting line, first at the finish.

* * *

Picture our friend, suddenly alone. Old friends have been banished; new ones exist behind a glass. For them, the Dream is still intact, the will and its rewards are boundless.

They are genuinely bewildered at his sorry state. What can the matter be?

. . .

He remained ill, progressively, for almost a year. Pneumonia, various infections, memory lapses. On occasion, to the panic of those behind the glass, he lost his bearings entirely.

A psychologist remained invincibly upbeat, assured him and his friends that all this is 'quite normal, in your case.'

But what 'normal' might mean, and what his precise 'case' might be, remained obscure. Or dare we say obscured? The fact was that no one, family or friends or doctors, would utter the awful truth.

. . .

He is in hospital, I visit him. Surgery is contemplated.

He and I dwell uneasily at the eye of a hurricane. We speak equably of a number of things; acquaintances, books, his business affairs. Life, he reports, goes reasonably well—in most respects.

Thus our civilized talk becomes a cosmetic falsehood, like paint on a corpse. It infects us with a sad bravado.

The truth hovering between is something else. No one of his affairs could, by painful stretch of fantasy, be called reasonable or well. Everything, life itself, is unreasonable and unwell.

Still, like the beleaguered entities we are, we chatter on, each guarding a shabby pretense; that the Dream (the alas and former Dream), is intact.

. . .

Something happens. An overcharged vein ruptures. The futility of this, my collusion, all thumps to a dead end. I think perversely, Why not press things a bit?

Thereupon: Jeremy, when am I to bring you Communion?

There is a stirring, almost a spasm in his limbs. Then the comeback.

'Why should I agree to that, just because I'm ill? I never wanted it when I was well.'

Then something of a counter stroke, even a sneer: 'Still, I suppose you're obliged to play your part, priest above all.'

I explode; his wall of cynicism, the near impossibility of breaching it.

A week later, the awful surgery was done; he was weak as the newborn. A wispy monotone reached my ears, plaintive and gentle.

Would I visit him and offer a prayer?

. . .

Prayer and anointing. How compassionate and tender the words! ' "My servant lies ill at home." And Jesus said, "I will come and heal him." '

Jeremy served me a warning beforehand: 'I'm going through with this as though I believed. Don't expect too much of me.'

Could he know how little most of us expect—of God, of one another? Minimal faith, retarded faith, half faith. Schizoid faith; one hand on the Gospel, the other stuck in the cultural sewer.

And then something else; faith, the crawling out.

. . .

'But the official answered, "Lord, I am not worthy to have you come under my roof. You have only to say the word, and my servant will be healed."'

He wept like a child. I held him, urged: Don't play superhuman. Rage if you want, fret and stew. If you get out of hand, we know enough to snarl back.

That brought a laugh, a shift of mood.

. . .

'Then Jesus said, "Go, it is done as you have believed." And the servant was healed at that moment.'

Priest: Let us pray for our brother, and for those who serve and care for him.

All: Hear our prayer.

I touch the forehead of Jeremy with the oil, and trace a cross.

Let us pray. Through this holy anointing may Christ our healer and brother bring you the grace of the Holy Spirit.

Lord Jesus you became one of us, to heal and save. Mercifully hear our prayer for the healing of our brother whom we anoint in your name.

There was a long silence. He murmured, 'I feel a power I have not known before.'

. . .

We were only at the beginning. Ahead were agony and false hope and illusory, ever weaker recovery.

There came too a slow shift in the attitude of his family.

They lost hope. Or rather, they lost that false hope that 'keeps going,' juggling the known truth.

I saw it in their faces, in the looks they bent his way. A new compassion arose, less bickering and banter.

Silence was taking form, they were trying silence as one tries a new element or an unsteady ground. They stepped timorously, breathed deeply.

Step by step, we were entrusting him to the Great Silence.

• • •

He plunged toward the end, into a source.

Standing at the edge, we wept; even as he reveled, clowned, cleansed himself, drowned and arose.

• • •

Dear Daniel:

You asked me recently if I would be interested in complementing your portrait of Jeremy with one of my own. Your suggestion took on an urgency despite the distance of three years. As a surviving relative, I was closest to him in his lifetime and stood by him at every stage of his illness. Although the events preceding Jeremy's death are still raw in my mind, and something akin to repulsion grips me whenever I summon them up, nonetheless, I offer these reflections out of fidelity to his memory. My contribution may help your readers grasp something of Jeremy's life, especially his journey through the dark valley of AIDS.

How does one isolate the mainspring of another's actions, how grasp the central motive? Like amateur scientists, we gather details, register cause and effect, construct a plausible theory. However astute the analysis, no one can claim to have penetrated another's core; we have only impressions to guide us towards clarity. What follows is one man's version.

When I replay my memories of Jeremy, I ask myself whether I sense some underlying cause or interconnecting link. You've pointed to the Dream of immortal youth, achievement and money. I cannot deny your description of what occupies many Americans. But I would supplement the Dream by including one other element which was fundamental to Jeremy's life: his relationship to Mitchell. This man was the center of Jeremy's universe around which business and family and friends were satellites. In his life with Mitch, Jeremy sought to combine sexuality, tenderness and friendship. What should have been a source of growth became, instead, a retardation. If the relationship grew, it did so by supplanting everything else. It ousted much of the past and set rigid boundaries for the present; while those who watched knew it boded ill for the future. If Jeremy's life was daily an either-or proposition, towards Mitch there was unconditional allegiance. It brooked no rivals. And what was true for Jeremy was true for Mitch. The symbiosis came full circle. I use the psychological term advisedly. This relationship had little to do with a healthy bonding based on distinction of persons. Mitch became Jeremy; Jeremy, Mitch. "We're in each other," Jeremy told me once with alarming candor; and I was reminded of that terrifying scene in Bronte's Wuthering Heights when Cathy confesses to Ellen, "I am Heathcliff." Without the Sacred as center, the relationship was made to carry impossible burdens. The posture of clinging and dependency precipitated constant bickering, even physical abuse—all aborted efforts to carve out individuality. In the end, it took a shared disease to separate them by death. Those who watched saw it coming with locomotive velocity. We were powerless to stop it.

In reflecting upon Jeremy's tragedy, which can be read as a story of obsessive love, I find present there what is endemic in the population: a yearning for some perfect emotional alliance, some towering other who represents all that is or can be; by definition, an image of eternity, of beatific fulfillment. This "absolutizing tendency"—to cite William Lynch's expression for it—is the longing for God in each of us now gone haywire in impossible romanticism. In a word, idolatry. If Jeremy violated any command of the Decalogue, it was not the Sixth or Ninth on the rostrum of shall-nots, but the First: I am the Lord, thy God; no strange gods before thee.

They were striking, Jeremy and Mitch: handsome, intelligent, funny, with boundless energy. They had given birth to a thriving business which they watched over like doting parents. And the business set unlimited boundaries for their exploits. Like Gilgamesh and Enkidu in the Sumerian epic, they went off together to conquer the world. Having youth and health on their side, they were, together, invincible. The heights were reached one evening at Studio One when the fruits of their labor flashed on the wall and the admiring crowds gloried in their success. It would not be long before our heroes were brought very low.

I do not want to prolong this story. It took AIDS and its onslaught to tease these two apart. Dying does that, for it's something we do alone. If love reaches across the gap, illness makes the other retreat still farther where no bridge can reach. Jeremy's dying decentralized the relationship with Mitch, who was himself critically ill. It was then that he turned to the Inner Guru and heard that 'still small voice' whose volume over the years had been reduced to a murmur. The golden calf of Human Love was smashed and the covenant ark returned to its central niche. Jeremy reached for the One who outwaits (outwits?) all human lovers. That providential Grace, of which Chesterton spoke in his admirable metaphor, had let Jeremy wander, then pulled him back with an unseen hook and 'a twitch upon the thread.'

How sad that in his lifetime we could not pull him up short and shake him to his senses. We coaxed and cajoled, cautioned and admonished. Nothing worked. The relationship overrode everything. In the end, only God was empowered to get a hearing, the Alone with the alone.

I miss Jeremy. For all the lopsidedness of his relationship, he made efforts at altruism, thoughtfulness and concern; at real giving and sharing. It came in spurts. It may be that the spurts, collected over a lifetime, became the torrent which in the end washed him clean.

As I held Jeremy, I remembered some lines from Merton's poem, "For My Brother: Reported Missing In Action, 1943," and prayed them:

> In the wreckage of your April Christ lies slain,
> And Christ weeps in the ruins of my spring;
> The money of Whose tears shall fall
> Into your weak and friendless hand,
> And buy you back to your own land:
> The silence of Whose tears shall fall
> Like bells upon your alien tomb.
> Hear them and come: they call you home.

In the hour of his death, Jeremy heeded the call and came home.

Julian Martell

EPILOGUE

FOR A SERVICE
OF PRAYER.
(DIGNITY; Miami,
July 26, 1987)

Mark 7: 24-30: Jesus rose and went away to the region of Tyre and Sidon. He entered a house, and would not have anyone know it. Yet he could not be hid. Immediately a woman, whose little daughter was possessed by an unclean spirit, heard of him; she came and fell down at his feet. Now the woman was a Greek, a Syrophoenician by birth. And she begged him to cast out the demon from her daughter. He said to her; Let the children first be fed, for it is not right to take the children's bread and cast it to the dogs. But she answered him, Yes, Lord; yet even the dogs under the table eat the children's crumbs that fall there. And he responded; For this saying you may go your way; the demon has left your daughter. And she went to her home, and found the child lying in bed, and the demon gone.

I commend this text to you, and to my own soul. Many of us have, we are told, for different reasons, something less than a human claim on the bread of Christ; which is to say, on his attentiveness, his response, his healing. Certain claims are neither large nor persuasive. What, after all, is the worth of a canine claim, proceeding as it does from a dog's life?

Indeed, to voice the claim, let alone insist on it, is considered a joke of sorts. The joke is often told, in ways diverse but unmistakable, by those on the inside track. Some claims are no larger than a crumb, no more persuasive than a dog's whine.

Those securely in possession, established where they sit—they are given to glances, words, slamming of doors in faces, such acts as might improve the occasion when a stray dog enters a banquet hall. Or a church.

Of more than passing interest is the harshness of Christ toward this mother. He seems bent, in contrast with other encounters with women, on humiliating her, making sport of her outcast condition.

Outcast she surely is, on at least two scores. She is a woman, and a non-Jew. Were she a Jewish woman, her status would be humiliating enough, as we learn from Torah and Christian testament. She would periodically be rendered unclean, unfit for worship, having little or no legal recourse or redress. Literally, as we are told on another occasion, she could be described as bent double under the burden of her humiliated legal and religious status.

But at very least, in such a hideous arrangement, a Jewish woman had a claim of sorts on salvation, a tradition of women—Jezebel, Deborah, Miriam, Judith, Anna—who surpassed gloriously the destiny to which they were condemned. Such women spoke up loud and clear, liberated themselves and others, sweetly deceived men, murdered even, seized a place in the history of their people.

. . .

But the woman who approaches Jesus is radically an outsider, from every point of view. She and her daughter are gentiles; in the awful words of the Savior, they are no better than dogs, and to be treated no differently.

A cruel word game indeed. With a measure of relief, one notes that he pursues it for only a moment or two. And she? She tolerates it; she must, for she is the suppliant. But for another reason too, she can be patient and attentive, and watch for her opening. In her own eyes she is a being of worth, a woman. As such, she needs no outside instruction as to her place in the world.

And if that instruction is offered (it has undoubtedly been offered before), and moreover, is deliberately cruel, well—she is skilled in letting such things come and go. This too will pass.

So she persists, listens. Christ may invoke an image of defeat and even of degradation; given her chance, she will turn his words around, to her own advantage.

I commend her tactic, her dogged persistence, to you and myself.

There are a few things in her favor; and by implication in our own. The One she seeks out for help also knows something, and will in time know much more, of the status of outcast. There is a strange congruence here, which time will reveal, between the woman and the reluctant healer. One day, Christ will be accounted a criminal bound for capital punishment, destined to be removed from this world. A malefactor, deprived of whose presence and provocation both church and state will undoubtedly be benefited.

It is unlikely in such times as we are enduring that you or I will win a serious hearing from the church, or from civil authority for that matter; each so strangely resembling the other in recoiling from such lives as we believe we are called to live.

Still, in this we can be at peace, even so troubled a peace as the times allow. The church remains for the present adamant: against serious peacemaking, against the gay community. But in these matters, each in its own way a matter of life and death, it cannot be said that the church speaks for Christ. It could even be said that the church speaks in contrariety to Christ.

In our story, the conduct of Christ is instructive. The woman enters the house, unannounced and uninvited. Christ chooses on the occasion to try her mettle. Where is faith, he implies, except in the testing of faith? Will she fold, will her face fall, hearing his vile image? Will she creep away like a very dog? Or will she stand her ground, rebut him, do him one better?

Obviously there is something at stake here; more than verbal jousting. A zen scene perhaps. The zen master offers a puzzle, a koan; the discipline is to unravel it—oftener than not, at great expense of time and effort.

But the woman is no raw novice in this business. Her wits have sharpened on the carborundum wheel of the world. She has heard the arguments before: who is to survive, who prosper, and who go under; arguments that do not invariably include the powerless and poor. She reads faces and eyes. The same faith that sent her in search of a healer is strong in her now, when all seems futile and she, it would seem, is dismissed.

She refuses to pack. Humiliated before others, regarded publicly as something less than human, an intruder, a dog fit only to be put to the chain or the door—she will not be cowed, she will turn the insult to her own advantage.

She will crack the code.

'If I am a dog,' (she grants the hideous premise for the moment—and her granting is a measure both of her humility and her sense of dignity)—'If in your eyes I am no more than a dog, you have by no means canceled my claim on your compassion. Can you not feel compassion even for a dog? Then do so.'

We think of the church, and the official treatment of many today; and then we think of Christ and the woman. We are struck by a contrast. The church rejects, ostracizes, places certain people beyond the pale; on a lifelong basis. This is an old story, and no one of us need hear it again. Biology, say the authorities, is destiny. Your biology is banned. Good luck with your destiny.

In one way or another we have all undergone it.

With Christ there is a different outlook, a different outcome. A more human humanism, one might say. Biology, he says in effect, is vocation. Your biology is welcome. Pursue your vocation.

Thus the zen master proposes an image that implies, as koans do, a tease, an insult, a puzzle, an obstacle, a test, a rejection. And the woman, on the moment, resolves the koan, turns aside the insult, passes the test brilliantly. And at her riposte, as Mark's Gospel tells, Jesus is lost in admiration. He gives in, heals the woman's child.

He is mastered by her sweetness and strength, the unbreakable spirit of a woman whose life had been a long eking from a sour root.

I love her spirit, and commend it to you. She is like a woman of Northern Ireland, or of South Africa—or of the South Bronx. A survivor, and how much more.

Consider her; a rotten culture, or a rotten religion (or both in conjunction of interest) have branded her: outsider, pariah, dog. Jesus echoes the insult, for the last time; only to wipe it away. She has entered a new covenant; 'in My friendship.' And the spirit of death is banished from her family.

What shall we name that quality of hers, a gift that makes her an ideal and model for the outsider? Courage? Persistence?

In any case, she will accept the stigma (for the last time) and turn it around. She rejects rejection, and so wins the day.

I do not know, any more than you, whether church authority will renounce its sinfulness, will at last heal and bind up those it has wounded so grievously. (And so will be healed and bound up, and acknowledge her own wounds.) I do not know. I confess that I am surer of your soul and mine than I am of such authority.

Of this I am certain: of our calling to holiness, our vocation to persist, in season and out, in the work of healing others, even as we seek healing for ourselves.

Let me comment briefly on the conclusion of the Gospel episode. The mother declares that her child is afflicted with a demon, an 'unclean spirit.' A strange diagnosis indeed. But Jesus has no quarrel with her words; in effect he agrees with her. And it is of that spirit, which the mother has sensed in possession of her child, a spirit alien and dangerous, enervating, arrogant, lethal, that the child is healed.

Biblically speaking, such 'spirits' are inevitably carriers of death, in all its analogues and metaphors. Indeed, if we are aware today of the spiritual plight, the 'other side' of our culture, Americans would appear afflicted in a way parallel to the child. The spirit of death haunts lives, institutions, churches.

We note with dismay the purveying of death, at home and in the world; not just physical death, which in comparison with other forms and disguises is indeed a far lesser evil. But I think of that 'second death' of which the Bible speaks; a spirit of death that freezes the soul; death of the heart, numbing of the mind, death to compassion, to a sense of the truth, to a sense of one another. And worse; the 'putting to death,' with malign intent and sour will, of human variety, of sexual and racial and religious variety, all that 'wet and wildness' celebrated by the poet, to the honor of the Creator.

Biblically speaking, healing is never accomplished by the powerful, by those in command. Indeed the Bible underscores the illness of wrong power, the spirit of control, of ego run amok. The conditions of these so afflicted were, but for the compassion of God, all but terminal.

Like many of you, I have been at the side of the dying during these terrible years; stood by our sisters and brothers, relatives, lovers, friends, as they lived out, generally with nobility and good grace, their last days.

One cannot but note, in the midst of such atrocious suffering, a strange irony. Many of the dying are freed, some speedily, some gradually, of cultural entanglements, obsessions, fears, violence, greed, moral numbing. In their dying, many surpass themselves; they succeeded in freeing others as well.

Thus in the strange irony of grace, physical death brings with it a splendid power, a sea change. The dying have been freed of the spirit of death, they have renounced the cultural illness. Hands once healed became, at the end, the hands of healers.

So we take heart. We commend the woman who quite simply, with all her heart, on behalf of someone she loved, refused to give up. We might think of her act as a 'forgiving persistence' toward Christ. We might also wish to ponder a kind of 'persistent forgiveness' toward the church.

The woman refuses and persists. And so prevails.

And so must we. And so shall we.

We must forgive, deepen our love, persist in our conviction that even the church can be redeemed from sin.

In so fulfilling our vocation, we ourselves are healed.

www.ingramcontent.com/pod-product-compliance
Lightning Source LLC
Chambersburg PA
CBHW062015220426
43662CB00010B/1344